BRADY

GERIATRIC NURSING ASSISTANT

BRADY
GERIATRIC
NURSING ASSISTANT

Advanced Training In Selected Competencies

Dorothy M. Witmer, R.N., C., Ed.D.
Health Occupations Teacher Educator
University of Nebraska-Lincoln

BRADY
A Prentice Hall Division
Englewood Cliffs, N.J. 07632

Library of Congress Cataloging-in-Publication Data

Witmer, Dorothy.
    The geriatric nursing assistant : advanced training in selected
competencies / Dorothy Witmer.
      p. cm.
    "A Brady book."
    ISBN 0-89303-707-9
    1. Geriatric nursing. 2. Nurses' aides. I. Title.
    [DNLM: 1. Allied Health Personnel—education. 2. Geriatric
Nursing—education. WY 18 W825g]
    RC954.W54 1990
    610.73 '65—dc20
    DNLM/DLC
    for Library of Congress   89-16386
                                                    CIP

Editorial/production supervision and
   interior design: **Diane Delaney/Julie Boddorf**
Cover design: **Ben Santora**
Cover photo: **Four by Five, Inc. (Tom Rosenthal/Superstock)**
Manufacturing buyer: **Dave Dickey**

 © 1990 by **Prentice-Hall, Inc.**
A Division of Simon & Schuster
Englewood Cliffs, New Jersey 07632

Printed in the United States of America

10 9 8 7 6 5 4 3 2 1

ISBN 0-89303-707-9

PRENTICE-HALL INTERNATIONAL (UK) LIMITED, *London*
PRENTICE-HALL OF AUSTRALIA PTY. LIMITED, *Sydney*
PRENTICE-HALL CANADA INC., *Toronto*
PRENTICE-HALL HISPANOAMERICANA, S.A., *Mexico*
PRENTICE-HALL OF INDIA PRIVATE LIMITED, *New Delhi*
PRENTICE-HALL OF JAPAN, INC., *Tokyo*
SIMON & SCHUSTER ASIA PTE. LTD., *Singapore*
EDITORA PRENTICE-HALL DO BRASIL, LTDA., *Rio de Janeiro*

DEDICATION

This book is dedicated to my mother,
Mary Josephine Abbott,
who, with her abiding faith
and abundant wisdom, instilled in me
courage and confidence to achieve
my goals, and to all residents
of nursing homes, who deserve dignity
and respect as they search
for peace and life satisfaction.

CONTENTS

PREFACE   *xiii*

ACKNOWLEDGEMENTS   *xvii*

1 *INTRODUCTION TO CARE OF THE ELDERLY*   *1*

Who Are the Elderly?   1
Geriatric Care as a Specialty: The Geriatric Health Care Team   2
Role and Responsibility of the Geriatric Nursing Assistant   5
Prerequisites for the Geriatric Nursing Assistant   9
A Philosophy of Care Giving   9
Key Points   10
Self-Check   10
Suggested Activities   11
Clinical Application   11

2 *THE AGING PROCESS*   *17*

Theories of Aging   18
The Aging Process: Expected Physiological Changes   19
The Aging Process: Expected Emotional and Social Changes   37
The Total Person: Needs Assessment   38
Key Points   40
Self-Check   41
Suggested Activities   41
Clinical Application   42

3 *SENSORY LOSSES OF AGING PEOPLE*   *47*

Impact of Sensory Losses   48
Sensory Losses and Techniques for Compensating   48
Key Points   66
Self-Check   66

Suggested Activities 67
Clinical Application 67

4 *ENVIRONMENTAL NEEDS OF THE ELDERLY*   73

Understanding the Nursing Home Environment 74
The Relationships and Effects of the Environment 74
Understanding the Environmental Needs of Residents 74
Key Points 78
Self-Check 79
Suggested Activities 79
Clinical Application 80

5 *THE NEWLY ADMITTED ELDERLY RESIDENT*   85

A Critical Time 86
Need for Family Involvement 86
Key Points 88
Self-Check 89
Suggested Activities 90
Clinical Application 90

6 *COMMUNICATION IN THERAPEUTIC RELATIONSHIPS*   93

The Humanizing Environment 94
Implementing the Philosophy of Care 94
Basic Foundations of Relationships 96
Verbal and Nonverbal Techniques of Communication 97
Barriers to Communication 98
The Benefits of Touch and Humor 101
Written Communications 105
Telephone Communications 106
Key Points 107
Self-Check 107
Suggested Activities 108
Clinical Application 108

7 *INFECTION CONTROL AND ACCIDENT PREVENTION*   115

Infection Control 115

Infection Control 115
Important Words to Understand 116
Special Considerations with the Elderly 118
Acquired Human Immunodeficiency Virus 122
Key Points 128
Self-Check 128
Suggested Activities 129
Clinical Application 129

Accident Prevention 129

Preventing Accidents 130

Falls of Residents 130

Incident Reports 133

Key Points 134

The Use of Restraining Devices 135

Reasons for Restraining Devices 135

Key Points 139

Assisting in Disaster Drill Procedures 140

Procedures in Case of a Fire 140

Procedures in Case of a Bomb Threat 147

Key Points 150

Self-Check 150

Suggested Activities 152

Clinical Application 152

8 SAFE POSITIONING, TRANSFERRING, TRANSPORTING 155

Special Considerations for Positioning the Elderly 156

Special Considerations When Transferring the Elderly 156

Transferring a Resident from Place to Place 168

Key Points 176

Self-Check 177

Suggested Activities 177

Clinical Application 178

9 NUTRITIONAL AND FLUID BALANCES 181

Meeting the Changes in the Digestive System that Affect
   Nutrition and Fluid Balances in the Elderly 182

The Basic Nutritional Requirements 182

The Choking Resident 189

Intravenous Feedings 200

Residents with Tubes: General Nursing Care 202

Key Points 206

Self-Check 207

Suggested Activities 207

Clinical Application 208

10 BLADDER AND BOWEL MANAGEMENT 215

Meeting Changes in the Urinary System that Affect Bladder
   Functioning in the Elderly 215

Meeting Changes in the Digestive System that Affect Bowel
   Functioning in the Elderly 217

Key Points 219

Self-Check 219

Suggested Activities 219

Clinical Application 220

11   *COMMON DISEASES AND DISABILITIES OF THE ELDERLY*   227

Alzheimer's Disease and Related Disorders:
Age-Related Changes 227

Alzheimer's Disease 228

Related Disorders 238

Key Points 240

Self-Check 241

Suggested Activities 242

Clinical Application 242

Cerebral Vascular Accidents: Age-Related Changes 242

Physical Changes Due to CVA 243

Emotional Changes Due to CVA 243

Key Points 246

Self-Check 246

Suggested Activities 247

Clinical Application 247

Diabetes Mellitus: Age-Related Changes 247

The Disease and its Course 248

Treatment 248

Key Points 250

Self-Check 251

Suggested Activities 251

Clinical Application 251

Cancer: Age-Related Changes 252

The Disease and its Course 252

Treatment 253

Key Points 254

Self-Check 254

Suggested Activities 255

Clinical Application 255

Arthritis: Age-Related Changes 255

The Disease and its Course 256

Treatment 257

Key Points 259

Self-Check 259

Suggested Activities 259

Clinical Application 259

Chronic Obstructive Pulmonary Disease:
Age-Related Changes 260

The Disease and its Course 260

Treatment 262

Key Points 262

Self-Check   263
Suggested Activities   263
Clinical Application   264

Cardiovascular Disease: Age-Related Changes 264

The Disease and its Course   264
Treatment   266
Key Points   271
Self-Check   271
Suggested Activities   272
Clinical Application   272

12 *GRIEVING, DYING, AND DEATH*   *287*

The Grieving Resident and Family Members   287
Hospice Programs   295
Care of the Person Who Dies   295
Key Points   297
Self-Check   297
Suggested Activities   298
Clinical Application   298

13 *SPECIAL CARE SERIES*   *299*

Nursing Assistant Responses for Residents with
   Tracheostomies   300
Key Points   301
Nursing Assistant Responses for Residents Receiving
   Oxygen   301
Key Points   304
Nursing Assistant Responses for Residents with Casts   304
Key Points   306
Nursing Assistant Responses for Residents in Traction   306
Key Points   307
Nursing Assistant Responses for Residents with Possible Drug
   Reaction   308
Key Points   309
Self-Check   309
Suggested Activities   310
Clinical Application   311

14 *REDUCING JOB-RELATED STRESS*   *323*

The Concept of Stress   323
Definitions of Terms Related to Stress   325
Coping   326
Stressors Related to the Job   327
Time Management   329
Key Points   333

Suggested Activities   334
Clinical Application   334

READING LIST   *335*
GLOSSARY   *337*
INDEX   *347*

PREFACE

The Geriatric Nursing Assistant has been written as an advanced learning program for the dedicated nursing assistant who wants to develop the special competencies needed in caring for the elderly. The person who chooses to enter this learning program is recognized for the experience gained after completion of a basic nursing assistant course of training. The geriatric nursing assistant program is also intended to provide a second level of training, allowing nursing assistants to advance in knowledge, skill, and leadership in caring for aging individuals.

The nursing assistant who cares for the elderly is a special person indeed. He or she recognizes that additional competencies are needed to meet the diverse needs of each elderly person/client. This textbook will help you become a competent *geriatric nursing assistant.* The need to develop skills specific to care of the elderly is greater now than ever before. The older population is increasing steadily. As the older population grows in number, those needing help with activities of daily living will also increase steadily. The number of nursing home residents is expected to increase accordingly.

The approach to learning in this textbook follows a competency-based format. The word competency means a performance which is worthwhile, done with ability and safety and for which an employer will pay. The competencies in this textbook have been identified by geriatric specialists who hire and supervise nursing assistants in geriatric settings. Some of the areas of competency normally taught in a basic program of nursing assistance have been repeated because of the need to give added importance in the care of the elderly. The elderly person will be called person, client, or resident. These words will be used interchangeably. Each unit of learning has been organized to include the following:

A terminal performance objective: which describes the major area of competency to be achieved for that unit.

Enabling objectives: which are competencies that will help you to accomplish the major competency. Each enabling competency can be referred to as a sub-competency.

Review section: a section which refers you to previously learned principles and knowledge. Review will provide background information for the topic under discussion.

Theoretical concepts: the currently recognized ideas which provide the reasons for the needed competencies.

Skill checklists: step by step procedures for performing skills.

Clinical applications: assignments which give instruction to the nursing assistant on how to directly apply the skills in each unit to clients or to the workplace. Clinical application of what is learned helps to develop competency in the appropriate skill.

Assignments or worksheets: forms which give directions for clinical applications.

Self-checks: questions which help the learner to evaluate his/her own learning.

Suggested Activities: additional learning opportunities that help nursing assistants to accomplish the objectives.

Key Points: summary statements which condense important points of each unit and reflect the philosophy of care the geriatric nursing assistant should adopt.

The competency-based approach to learning allows the nursing assistant to complete the learning of one competency before moving on to the next. The units address the three areas that nursing assistants must develop in order to be competent: psychomotor (performance), cognitive (knowledge), and affective (attitudes). By taking advantage of the various learning activities provided in the text, the nursing assistant will develop in these three areas of competency.

Problem solving: Throughout the textbook are geriatric nursing assistant responses for clients who experience one, two, or many needs or problems. Each client is unique in his or her reactions to these needs or problems. The responses provided by the geriatric nursing assistant should be the result of the problem-solving process. The problem-solving process in the profession of nursing is called the "nursing process." Although the geriatric nursing assistant does not have the same responsibility as the professional nurse, the steps of the nursing process can help the assistant in developing a systematic method for helping the professional nurse with problem solving. The steps in the nursing process and the related activities which can be done by the geriatric nursing assistant follow.

Professional Nursing Activities in the Nursing Process	Geriatric Nursing Assistant Activities in the Nursing Process
These are accomplished by the registered nurse.	Activities performed by nursing assistants consistent with their scope of allowable activities.
1. *ASSESSMENT* Collection of data from many sources (client, family, clinical procedures) and arriving at needs/ problems.	1. Gathering of information through communication and observation of elderly clients; taking vital signs; reporting any changes, positive or negative, about the

2. *NURSING DIAGNOSIS*
A statement which indicates a client's response that is actually or potentially unhealthy and can be helped by nursing actions.

3. *PLANNING*
Determining nursing actions to be taken to help resolve needs/problems and achieve goals mutually agreed upon by nurse and client.

4. *INTERVENTION/IMPLEMENTATION*
Putting the actions into practice. Involving the client in self-care as much as possible.

5. *EVALUATION*
Determining progress or lack of progress toward goals. May mean reassessment and renewing the process.

client. Consider all body systems and the "total" person when noting positive or negative changes in each person.

2. Identifying needs and problems. These are conclusions drawn after gathering information.

3. Arriving at geriatric nursing assistant actions which may be possible solutions to the problem.

4. Applying the geriatric nursing assistant actions to help resolve the problem or satisfy the need.

5. Evaluating whether the nursing actions satisfied the need or resolved the problem. If the problem was not resolved, what other actions are necessary? Was the problem identified correctly? If not, go back to step one. The problem-solving nursing process is continuous and cyclical. It is used over and over again with daily care of the client.

These steps will help you think about how to respond uniquely to each individual in helping the individual to satisfy needs and to resolve problems which interfere with daily functioning. The process is applied over and over again as clients experience interference in performing independently.

You are encouraged to use the problem-solving process, the nursing process, in responding to the clinical applications given in this textbook. *Refer back to this reading with each clinical application that requests problem solving in situations with the elderly.*

ACKNOWLEDGEMENTS

This book is the result of support and encouragement of many people. The original work began during research in pursuit of a doctural degree at the University of Idaho. Deep appreciation for the necessary guidance during that time is extended to Dr. Cleve Taylor, Dr. James Bikkie, Dr. Doris Williams, and Dr. Zeph Foster. Assistance was received from members of the geriatric advisory committee, who identified the competencies for advanced training and reviewed the original manuscript: geriatric nursing practitioners Susan Acee and Susan McDermott; nursing home administrator Gary Bermeosolo; geriatrician Dr. Barry Cusak; supervisor of Health Occupations Sandra Davis; directors of nursing Bonnie Gholson, Delta Holloway, and Sally Johnson; and nursing home staff nurse Mary Stevens. Many nursing assistants also contributed by participating in surveys and in training using content that became part of this book. Numerous residents in nursing homes contributed to the inspiration and determination needed to bring the writing to its conclusion. Special acknowledgement and thanks are due to Leigh Mann, student assistant, who helped with typing the manuscript, and to Diane Delaney and Julie Boddorf for their excellent editorial assistance. However, without the love and support of my children, Jody, Joe, Kathy, and Steve, this book may never have been written.

1 *INTRODUCTION TO CARE OF THE ELDERLY*

TERMINAL PERFORMANCE OBJECTIVE

Assess yourself as a care giver and team member in the role of a geriatric nursing assistant.

Enabling Objectives

1. Use previously learned nursing assistant skills in the role of nursing assistant.
2. Participate as a geriatric health care team member.
3. Define the term *elderly*.
4. Identify members of the geriatric health care team.
5. Describe the difference between the basic nursing assistant and the geriatric nursing assistant.
6. Describe a philosophy of care for the elderly that is holistic and humanistic.
7. Assess yourself as a care giver and team member.

REVIEW SECTION

The topics you should review with the instructor are the health care team members, role and responsibilities (legal, ethical, employee) of the nursing assistant, and patient rights.

WHO ARE THE ELDERLY?

The *elderly* as a group in our society are generally classified as those 65 years of age and older. This is the age designated in the 1935 federal Social Security Act as the anticipated age of retirement. With the passage of the Social Security Act, persons 65 years of age and older received money to replace the money they had received when they were working. The availability of this retirement money encouraged many people to open homes to take in the elderly. As these people needed health care, the owners of the homes added nurses and soon the homes were designated as "nursing homes." Many owners were retired nurses; however, they did not consider themselves to be "geriatric nurses" as we know the title today.

Certainly, not everyone who reaches 65 should be considered "elderly." Each of you probably has relatives or neighbors 65 or older who continue to work outside the home and/or are very active in the community. On the other hand, there are people in their forties and fifties who seem very old to us because of chronic disease and lack of energy. It is obvious that chronological age, the number of years one has lived, has little to do with whether one feels old or elderly.

Various researchers have used different categories in assigning years to define the young-old, the old, the old-old, and the very old-old. With the current predictions, we can expect people to be living much longer and therefore, there will be more old-old and very old-old people in our society. The following list gives some of the years assigned to each category:

Young-old	55 to 75
Old	76 to 80
Old-old	81 to 90
Very old-old	91 to 100

People over 75 years are the fastest-growing segment of our population. According to a 1980 U.S. Census Bureau Report, by the year 2000, we can expect to have a population of 36 million people over the age of 65. There will be approximately 13 million people 85 and older by the year 2040. It is the old-old and very-old groups who will require the most assistance with activities of daily living. Many will probably need to be in a nursing home at least part of their advancing years.

It is important for the geriatric nursing assistant to remember that growing older is part of living. Of the aging populations, 95 percent live independently or fairly independently: with relatives, friends, or in retirement homes. The 5 percent of the elderly in nursing homes sometimes gives a distorted picture of the older population. Many 80- and 90-year-old people do quite well on their own.

GERIATRIC CARE AS A SPECIALTY: THE GERIATRIC HEALTH CARE TEAM

Geriatric care is slowly being recognized as a specialty similar to areas such as pediatrics (care of children) and obstetrics (care of expectant mothers). In the field of nursing, advances have been faster than in any other health care area. In 1961, a committee of the American Nurses Association recommended that there be a specialty group of geriatric nurses. The first group of nurses met in the spring of 1962 to form the Conference Group on Geriatric Nursing. In June 1966, the American Nurses Association developed a division of geriatric nursing practice. Standards to guide nursing practice were developed later. Today this division has grown to be recognized as an area of specialty training for nurses.

Physicians in the United States have been slower than nurses to recognize geriatrics as a specialty area. Today the specialty designation for physicians is the term *geriatrician*. Physicians who specialize are growing in number with the increase in geriatric study in the medical education curriculum.

Members of the geriatric health care team have not changed in title; however, their training should include the differences in care and approaches to rehabilitation needed for aging individuals. Everyone in health care working with elderly people should have special education in geriatrics. Numerous centers have been developed throughout the United States to train and educate professional and nonprofessional workers in the needs of elderly people. The geriatric health care team (Figures 1.1 and 1.2) includes, but is not limited to, the the following members:

Geriatrician: Physician who is a specialist in the diagnosis and treatment of the elderly.

Nursing care team:

geriatric nurse practitioner (GNP), a registered nurse who has advanced training in diagnosis, assessment, and treatment of elderly clients. The GNP works in collaboration with and under the supervision of the physician and participates as a member of the nursing care team.

registered nurses (R.N.s) and *licensed practical nurses* (L.P.N.'s), who take advanced training in care of the elderly.

geriatric nursing assistants, who take advanced training in nursing the elderly after completing basic nursing assistant training.

Physical therapist: Professional who concentrates on the maintenance and rehabilitation of the musculoskeletal systems.

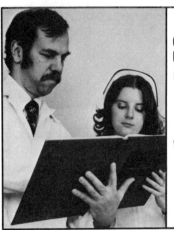

GERIATRIC NURSE PRACTITIONER

Registered nurse who has taken advanced training in geriatrics and a preceptorship with a physician who specializes in geriatrics

Works under supervision of a physician. Assists with assessment, diagnosis, and treatment. Contributes to the nursing care plan

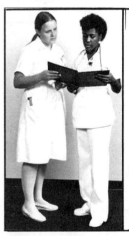

PROFESSIONAL REGISTERED NURSE

Four-year university education with a bachelor's degree

or

Two-year junior or community college education with an associate degree

or

Three-year diploma from a hospital nursing school

and

Passed state board examinations

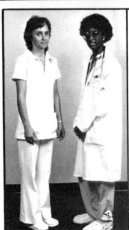

LICENSED PRACTICAL NURSE (LPN)

or

LICENSED VOCATIONAL NURSE (LVN)

One-year training program

Passed state board examinations

PLPN—Pharmaceutical Licensed Practical Nurse is one who administers drugs or medications after taking a special course and passing a special examination

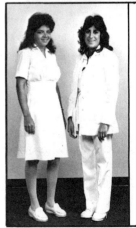

**NURSING ASSISTANT
NURSING AIDE
NURSE'S AIDE
NURSE'S ASSISTANT
HOME HEALTH AIDE
HOME HEALTH ASSISTANT
GERIATRIC AIDE
GERIATRIC ASSISTANT
ORDERLY
NURSING ATTENDANT**

All are names used for the non-professional worker who, under the direction and supervision of the registered nurses, carries out basic bedside nursing functions

Figure 1.1. Nursing care team.

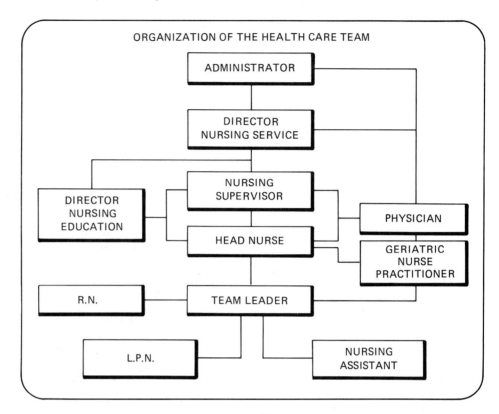

ORGANIZATION OF THE HEALTH CARE TEAM

Figure 1.2. Health care team.

Occupational therapist: Professional who concentrates on rehabilitation of the client to perform activities of daily living.

Speech therapist: Professional who concentrates on rehabilitation of speech.

Audiologist: Professional who specializes in hearing.

Recreational therapist: Professional who concentrates on recreational and social activities.

Dietician: Professional who concentrates on nutritional and dietary needs.

Other professionals and paraprofessionals are employed to assist with the plan of care of an elderly client (Figure 1.3). Each of these people are considered as part of the team, although they may not be in the facility at all times. The ophthalmologist and optometrist are eye specialists. The podiatrist deals with foot problems. The dentist is concerned with dental problems and age-related dental disorders. These professionals often have assistants who are less skilled but are trained as paraprofessionals in the specific area of service.

The purpose of the geriatric health care team is to work together with the elderly client and his or her family members to provide the best kind of care possible. The team members operate to achieve goals mutually set with the client and the significant members of the client's family. The goals and actions required to achieve them compose the client's plan of care. The geriatric nursing assistant is responsible as part of the nursing care team to assist in accomplishing the determined goals.

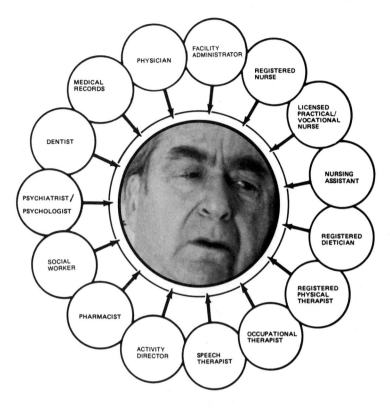

Figure 1.3.   Client–centered health care.

ROLE AND RESPONSIBILITY OF THE GERIATRIC NURSING ASSISTANT

At the beginning of this unit you were reminded to review the role of the nursing assistant with regard to legal, ethical, and employee responsibilities. As a geriatric nursing assistant, these areas of responsibility do not change. You work under the supervision of a registered nurse who may choose to delegate the supervision to a licensed practical nurse.

As a geriatric nursing assistant, you provide the greatest amount of care to elderly clients. It has been estimated that nursing assistants provide at least 90 percent of the care to residents in nursing homes. Because of their advanced training, geriatric nursing assistants are able to assume a leadership role and set an example to other untrained nursing assistants. Your contribution to the care of the elderly is more meaningful and valuable because of advanced training that other nursing assistants do not have. You can contribute to improved function and independence of each client. Your duty areas and tasks do not change. However, the special training in geriatric care helps the geriatric nursing assistant to individualize care and to look for innovative ways to assist elderly clients to achieve optimal health. Remember to recognize the rights of clients and to protect them as you give care (see Patient's Bill of Rights, p. 6).

A sample job description is provided in Figure 1.4. This will help you further identify the differences between the basic nursing assistant and one who has special training in care of the elderly.

The job description emphasizes the individuality of the aging person. Too often the elderly have been stereotyped as being very much alike, yet the op-

Patient's Bill of Rights

These patients' rights, policies and procedures ensure that each patient admitted to the facility at least is:

- Fully informed, as evidenced by the patient's written acknowledgment, prior to or at the time of admission and during his stay, of these rights and of all rules and regulations governing patient conduct and responsibilities;

- Fully informed, prior to or at the time of admission and during stay, of services available in the facility, and of related charges including any charges for services not covered under titles XVIII or XIX of the Social Security Act, or not covered by the facility's basic per diem rate;

- Fully informed, by a physician, of his medical condition unless medically contraindicated (as documented, by a physician, in his medical record), by a physician, in his medical record, and is afforded the opportunity to participate in the planning of his medical treatment and to refuse to participate in experimental research;

- Transferred or discharged only for medical reasons, or for his welfare or that of other patients, or for non-payment for his stay (except as prohibited by titles XVIII or XIX of the Social Security Act), and is given reasonable advance notice to ensure orderly transfer or discharge, and such actions are documented in his medical record;

- Encouraged and assisted, throughout his period of stay, to exercise his rights as a patient and as a citizen, and to this end may voice grievances and recommend changes in policies and services to facility staff and/or to outside representatives of his choice, free from restraint, interference, coercion, discrimination, or reprisal;

- May manage his personal financial affairs or be given, at least quarterly, an accounting of financial transactions made on his behalf should the facility accept his written delegation of this responsibility for any period of time, in conformance with State law;

- Free from mental and physical abuse, and free from chemical and (except in emergencies) physical restraints except as authorized in writing by a physician for a specified and limited period of time, or when necessary to protect the patient from injury to himself or to others;

- Assured confidential treatment of his personal and medical records, and may approve or refuse their release to any individual outside the facility, except, in case of his transfer to another health care institution, or as required by law or third-party payment contract;

- Treated with consideration, respect, and full recognition of his dignity and individuality, including privacy in treatment and in care for his personal needs;

- Not required to perform services for the facility that are not included for therapeutic purposes in his plan of care;

- Free to associate and communicate privately with persons of his choice, and send and receive his personal mail unopened, unless medically contraindicated (as documented by his physician in his medical record);

- Free to meet with, and participate in activities of social, religious, and community groups at his discretion, unless medically contraindicated (as documented by his physician in his medical record);

- Free to retain and use his personal clothing and possessions as space permits, unless to do so would infringe upon rights of other patients, and unless medically contraindicated (as documented by his physician in his medical record); and

- If married, is assured privacy for visits by his/her spouse; if both are in-patients in the facility, they are permitted to share a room, unless medically contraindicated (as documented by the attending physician in the medical record).

These rights may only be denied under special circumstances, such as when a resident is judged to be medically incapable of understanding these rights *by the attending physician* or through the legal system.

A SAMPLE JOB DESCRIPTION

Occupational Title: Geriatric Nursing Assistant

General Description: The Geriatric Nursing Assistant has completed a formal course of training in basic nursing assisting skills and an advanced program of training in the special competencies needed to care for the aging person. The Geriatric Nursing Assistant has a thorough knowledge of the aging process, the special needs of the aging person, and the application of nursing responses to meet those needs.

Supervision: The Geriatric Nursing Assistant is supervised by a Registered Nurse or a Licensed Practical Nurse, whoever is designated as the charge nurse.

Major Duties and Tasks: The Geriatric Nursing Assistant works as a cooperative geriatric nursing care team member in meeting the needs and goals of each resident as written on the nursing care plan. He or she communicates effectively with team members and residents, recognizes the uniqueness of each resident, and applies principles of restorative and rehabilitative nursing in caring for each resident. Specific tasks include: the promotion of independence and wellness in each resident in the performance of activities of daily living, the specific tasks of personal care to residents who require them, and assistance with duties that help the unit to operate harmoniously. The characteristics that distinguish the Geriatric Nursing Assistant from others without specialized training are: the ability to communicate effectively to discover residents' specific needs; the ability to assist residents and team members to solve problems and to satisfy those needs; the ability to approach each resident in a holistic manner, recognizing the many dimensions that each person has. In addition, the Geriatric Nursing Assistant has the ability to apply innovative methods to help each resident have a self-fulfilling life. He or she uses continuing education as a means of improving care.

Figure 1.4. A sample job description.

posite is true. The physical characteristics of aging are similar, but the personality and makeup of aging people are as different as those of any other age group. Following is a care-giver checklist that can be used for self-evaluation of approaches to the elderly.

CARE GIVER CHECKLIST

Directions: Circle the letter if it applies to you.

1. Recognizing the elderly client as a unique person with individual characteristics, abilities, and interests.
    a. I identify myself by name to the client, visitors, and family members.
    b. I address the client by his or her preferred name.
    c. I assist clients to become oriented to the facility.
    d. I learn all I can about clients' interests, lifestyle, and social, cultural, and religious background in order to understand, and anticipate, their needs.

    e. I encourage the client to make decisions and choices as much as possible.

    f. I encourage the client to do as much as he or she can safely do.

    g. I am conscious of each client's need to receive empathetic, individualistic care.

    h. I respect the client's privacy by knocking on the door before entering, by pulling privacy curtains, and by preventing overexposure of body parts.

    i. I assist each client in making the best possible appearance.

    j. I use language that is respectful and understood by the client and family members.

    k. I provide for clients to be alone with loved ones.

    l. I safeguard each client's possessions.

    m. I am patient and kind with clients whose mental ability is declining.

2. Giving skilled care

    a. I anticipate the client's need for prevention and safety in all care given.

    b. I am competent in all personal care skills.

    c. I collaborate with the client in promoting self-care, restoration, and rehabilitation.

    d. I collaborate with the geriatric health care team in reaching mutual goals established with the client.

    e. I continually search for new ways to help clients who show declining mental ability.

    f. I am unhurried in my care.

3. Providing a humanizing environment

    a. I listen attentively to client's feelings as well as words.

    b. I am warm and accepting regardless of the client's hostility, anger, and denial.

    c. I act on behalf of the client's rights.

    d. I provide clients with a sense of equality and value their participation in daily activities.

    e. I remember that the client's home is now the institution and I try to make it a place of comfort and security.

4. Providing reality assurance and reality orientation

    a. I do not give false hopes to clients when there is doubt.

    b. I provide comfort measures when a client is uncomfortable.

    c. I observe and report immediately any client who is in pain and then follow up to be sure that pain is relieved.

    d. I help the client talk about fears and stay close when he or she is apprehensive.

    e. I use the techniques of reality orientation to help clients who will benefit by them.

    f. I give extra attention to new clients to help them adjust because I know that this is a difficult time for them.

5. Fulfilling responsibilities as an employee

    a. I desire to work with the elderly.

    b. I maintain good physical and mental health, leaving any personal problems at home.

    c. I know my job and what is expected of me.

    d. I am responsible for my own actions.

    e. I arrive for work on time.

    f. I notify my employer as soon as possible of illness or circumstances preventing my arrival at work.

    g. I conserve energy, equipment, and supplies.

    h. I work as an effective team member.
    i. I maintain a proper dress code.
    j. I avoid selling products to clients for additional income.
    k. I attend continuing education programs to improve myself and my competency in caring for the elderly.

PREREQUISITES FOR THE GERIATRIC NURSING ASSISTANT

The geriatric nursing assistant is expected to have completed a basic course of training in nursing assisting. The suggested prerequisites for entering specialty training as an advanced geriatric nursing assistant are listed below. These prerequisites have been verified as being essential to performance in the program and on the job. Entry into the program without one or more of these prerequisites may affect a learner's chances of success in the training program and on the job.

A. Physical abilities, traits, or characteristics
    1. Strong back and legs
    2. Able to assist in moving a person weighing 200 pounds
    3. Able to move quickly and to walk distances
B. Previously learned skills
    1. Completed an approved nursing assisting program of basic nursing skills, *or*
    2. Have sufficient knowledge and experience to be successful in a basic nursing assisting course
C. Previously learned knowledge
    1. Able to read and comprehend the instructions given in this program, which are similar to but considered to be in greater depth than those of a basic curriculum
D. Previously acquired attitudes
    1. Enjoys and desires working with the aging
    2. Believes in humanistic approaches to the aging which will help to restore their potential

A PHILOSOPHY OF CARE GIVING

The geriatric nursing assistant performs a very significant role in the care-giving process. Because the geriatric nursing assistant provides the greatest care, it is essential that care be based on a philosophy that is holistic and humanistic (Figure 1.5). To provide care in a holistic way means that the care giver accepts the fact that each elderly person has unique characteristics, abilities, and interests. Each elderly person is recognized as having a lifetime of experiences different from those of any other person. The combination of these experiences have influenced the person physically, psychologically, socially, and environmentally. Everyone is different and requires at least a variation in response that is unique to that person. When the care giver provides care in keeping with the uniqueness required for each person, holistic care is being given.

    The geriatric nursing assistant who provides humanistic care recognizes the dimensions of humanness. These dimensions have been described by many authors, including Bowker and Howard. The dimensions of humanistic care are discussed in more detail later in the book, but a summary is provided here. Humanistic care includes: respect, dignity, and a sense of worth in care giving; providing choices to the extent possible; involving the client in the care planning

THE HELPING RELATIONSHIP

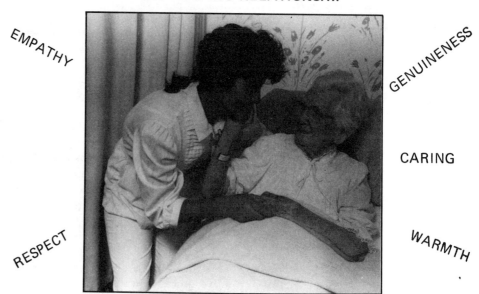

EMPATHY

GENUINENESS

CARING

RESPECT

WARMTH

Figure 1.5.   The helping relationship.

process; addressing the client as an equal, avoiding a subservient manner; and providing opportunity for the client to have some control over his or her life. The geriatric nursing assistant who incorporates these dimensions of humanness in the care-giving process is providing care in a humanistic way.

KEY POINTS

1. Growing old is another phase of living.
2. Each person ages differently and is unique in his or her own individuality; therefore, the basic retirement age of 65 years provided in the Social Security Act of 1935 does not define a person as "old."
3. The geriatric nursing assistant can make a positive difference in the life of each client to whom he or she gives care. Self-assessment will help to identify strengths and weaknesses as a care giver.
4. It is necessary to adopt a philosophy that provides holistic and humanistic approaches if quality care is to be given.
5. The geriatric nursing assistant is an important part of a geriatric health care team and can effectively work with other team members to assist clients in achieving goals on which the client and team members mutually agree.

SELF-CHECK

1. What federal act contributed to "defining" the age when people are considered old? What age was assigned to the elderly by this act?
2. Discuss the statement: "You are only as old as you feel."
3. How does the role of geriatric nursing assistant differ from that of a person who finished a basic program of nursing assisting?
4. What kind of attitude is desirable for the geriatric nursing assistant?

5. Identify four health care team members of different disciplines who work together to carry out a plan of care for a person with left-sided paralysis.
6. Using the care-giver checklist, identify five characteristics of the geriatric nursing assistant.
7. Describe a philosophy of geriatric care, and how is it applied in daily nursing assistant activities?

SUGGESTED ACTIVITIES

1. Request to participate in multidisciplinary team meetings about clients for whom you give care.
2. Speak with family members about activities a withdrawn person once enjoyed. Look for innovative ways to involve that person; consult with team members for advice and assistance.
3. Talk with a nursing assistant who is new to the job and to one who has been caring for the elderly for 2 to 3 years. Ask them to answer the self-check questions. Discuss in class what differences you found.
4. Review the list of patient rights and list the ones you feel are often disregarded. What can you do to correct any violations?

CLINICAL APPLICATION

It is recommended that two clinical applications be completed for this unit:

1. The worksheet on the health care team. This will help to make you aware of the variety of contributions from people on the health care team.
2. An evaluation by your supervisor, using the care-giver checklist, of your strengths and weaknesses in performance, so that you can begin a plan for self-improvement.

WORKSHEET

Health Care Team Members Involved in Resident's Care

Resident: _____   Diagnosis: _____
            (first name only)

Directions: In the left column under "Team Member," write in the name of the team member; start with yourself. In the right column under "Responsibility to . . . ," write in what the team member does for the resident.

Team Member	Responsibility to Resident and Resident's Plan of Care
1. Nursing Assistant	
2.	
3.	
4.	

WORKSHEET

Care-Giver Checklist

Directions: Circle the letter if it applies to you.
1. Recognizing the elderly client as a unique person with individual characteristics, abilities, and interests
   a. I identify myself by name to the client, visitors, and family members.
   b. I address the client by his or her preferred name.
   c. I assist clients to become oriented to the facility.
   d. I learn all I can about clients' interests, lifestyle, and social, cultural, and religious background in order to understand and anticipate their needs.
   e. I encourage the client to make decisions and choices as much as possible.
   f. I encourage the client to do as much as he/she can safely do.
   g. I am conscious of each client's need to receive empathetic, individualistic care.
   h. I respect the client's privacy by knocking on the door before entering, by pulling privacy curtains, and by preventing overexposure of body parts.
   i. I assist each client in making the best possible appearance.
   j. I use language that is respectful and understood by the client and family members.
   k. I provide for clients to be alone with loved ones.
   l. I safeguard each client's possessions.
   m. I am patient and kind with clients whose mental ability is declining.
2. Giving skilled care
   a. I anticipate the client's need for prevention and safety in all care given.
   b. I am competent in all personal care skills.
   c. I collaborate with the client in promoting self-care, restoration, and rehabilitation.
   d. I collaborate with the geriatric health care team in reaching mutual goals established with the client.
   e. I continually search for new ways to help clients who show declining mental ability.
   f. I am unhurried in my care.
3. Providing a humanizing environment
   a. I listen attentively to client's feelings as well as words.
   b. I am warm and accepting regardless of the client's hostility, anger, and denial.
   c. I act on behalf of the client's rights.
   d. I provide clients with a sense of equality and value their participation in daily activities.
   e. I remember that the client's home is now the institution and I try to make it a place of comfort and security.
4. Providing reality assurance and reality orientation
   a. I do not give false hopes to clients when there is doubt.
   b. I provide comfort measures when a client is uncomfortable.

c. I observe and report immediately any client who is in pain and then follow up to be sure that pain is relieved.

d. I help the client talk about fears and stay close when he or she is apprehensive.

e. I use the techniques of reality orientation to help clients who will benefit by them.

f. I give extra attention to new clients to help them adjust because I know that this is a difficult time for them.

5. Fulfilling responsibilities as an employee

a. I desire to work with the elderly.

b. I maintain good physical and mental health, leaving any personal problems at home.

c. I know my job and what is expected of me.

d. I am responsible for my own actions.

e. I arrive for work on time.

f. I notify my employer as soon as possible of illness or circumstances preventing my arrival at work.

g. I conserve energy, equipment, and supplies.

h. I work as an effective team member.

i. I maintain a proper dress code.

j. I avoid selling products to clients for additional income.

k. I attend continuing education programs to improve myself and my competency in caring for the elderly.

2 *THE AGING PROCESS*

TERMINAL PERFORMANCE OBJECTIVE

Given information about the aging person and the aging process, and a worksheet, use the problem-solving process to complete a needs assessment of an aging person and provide geriatric nursing assistant responses to help meet the identified needs and to help the person to achieve optimal functioning.

Enabling Objectives

1. Describe three theories of aging currently believed to contribute to the aging process.
2. Identify three age-related changes that occur in each of the following systems of the body: integumentary, circulatory, respiratory, muscular, skeletal, digestive, endocrine, urinary, reproductive, and nervous.
3. Provide five geriatric nursing assistant responses for each of the body systems listed in this unit.
4. List the five levels of need outlined by Abraham Maslow and explain why some older people have difficulty satisfying them.
5. Explain three social and three emotional changes that occur in the older person's life.
6. Complete a needs assessment of a selected older person using the problem-solving worksheet provided in this unit, and describe the geriatric nursing assistant responses that will help to meet those needs.

REVIEW SECTION

The topics to be reviewed with the instructor are normal anatomy and basic physiology of the body systems and emotional and social needs common to all people.

THEORIES OF AGING

A theory is a belief or reasonable set of principles based on fact that is offered to explain various phenomena. A theory is often an unproven assumption. The theories presented here are somewhat controversial.

Many scientific investigators have been trying to discover why we grow old. Some of these theories are described briefly in this unit to inform you of the kind of research that is being conducted. An explanation of how aging may occur will help you to understand the physical and mental changes that can be seen in older people. The aging process is still a mystery. Why the aging process occurs differently in different individuals at various ages has not been explained satisfactorily in the scientific world. At this time, why we age is still very much under investigation.

The *free-radical theory* is one that is gaining in popularity. Free radicals are pieces of molecules that break off from their original molecule and become attached to other molecules, thereby causing changes and damage. The free-radical theory is tied to the cell. Scientists believe that free radicals penetrate body cells and cause damage. Some researchers have found that vitamins E, A, and C protect the cells from free-radical damage. Free radicals occur in the body from the food we eat and also enter the body from the environment. The best known external source to add free radicals to the body is smog. If the free-radical theory is correct, watching what kind of food we eat and staying away from smog should help protect us from the cell damage and cell breakdown that occur in aging.

The *cross-link theory* is based on the linkage of several molecules that normally are separate. The other name for this idea is the *collagen theory*. Collagen is normally present in about 25 to 30 percent of body protein. It is responsible for maintaining structural support to body tissues such as skin, tendons, bone, muscle, and heart. Scientists believe that collagen cross-links with chemicals of the body such as lipids and carbohydrates to cause changes. The cross-linkage occurs more rapidly between the ages of 30 and 50 years. Visible results of the linkage are most prominent in the skin, which often becomes dry, begins to sag, and loses its softness. Other effects of these changes are seen in the teeth, which may loosen; in loss of strength in arterial walls; and in decreased efficiency of the stomach and intestinal linings. It is believed that restriction of caloric intake helps to slow the cross-linkage process.

The *immunological theory* of aging is another widely accepted theory. Scientists believe that as a person grows older the cells of the immune system become more diverse and are less able to regulate themselves. As the regulation of the cell decreases, cells that are normal to the body are identified as enemies and are actually attacked by the immune system. The theory has been associated with diseases such as cancer and diabetes mellitus in older adults. Scientists do not agree on whether the immune system is deficient because of aging or whether the deficient immune system causes aging. Investigations are under way to alter the immune system of older adults to prevent the complications and diseases that result from a poor immune system.

The *programmed aging theory* and the *biologic clock theory* are often considered to be the same. This theory means that aging is controlled by genes. It sees the genes as containing the limits for the rate and time that a member of a species, in this case the human species, will die.

Other theories about why aging occurs have not been discussed here. The theories presented will give some idea as to why aging occurs. The information provided should increase our understanding of what scientists are trying to discover about the aging process and may one day be of benefit.

THE AGING PROCESS: EXPECTED PHYSIOLOGICAL CHANGES

As a person ages, the first noticeable signs are physical: graying hair, wrinkled skin, slower pace of walking, and less physical activity. Each person ages differently and at different times. Some people seem "old" at 50 years, while others defy their chronological age and seem very young and active at 80 or 90.

Many factors contribute to how people age. Lifestyles, acute and chronic diseases, accidents, emotional stress, and poor environmental conditions contribute to a person's aging process. In general, as one ages, the body organs decrease in number of cells and in functioning ability. On the following pages are shown drawings of the body systems with the age-related changes, consequences of changes, and the responses that geriatric nursing assistants can provide to assist elderly clients with those changes.

Integumentary System: The Skin (Figure 2.1)

Changes	*Consequences of Changes*
Decreased number of cells	Skin becomes dry and fragile
Decreased moisture	Less tolerance for the sun
Thinning of layers of skin	Increased susceptibility to infection
Connective tissue becomes rigid	
Decreased elasticity	Decreased tolerance to heat and cold
Decreased amount of body hair	
Nails become dry and brittle	May lead to heat exhaustion (hyperthermia) or hypothermia (unsafe lowering of body temperature)
Decreased subcutaneous fat	
Decreased blood flow	
Decreased perspiration	Skin tears and bruises easily

Geriatric nursing assistant responses   The following actions can be taken by the geriatric nursing assistant to compensate for skin changes that occur in older clients.

1. Use lubricating lotion in bath water rather than soaps, which cause drying. If soap is used, rinse the skin thoroughly.
2. Pat the skin dry; do not rub roughly.
3. Apply lotions to bony, prominent body parts such as elbows, shoulders, hips, sacral area, and heals, using massage strokes, especially after bathing and when turning the client in bed.
4. Keep the client covered as much as possible during bathing procedures. Assist the client to dress quickly after bathing, and to dress appropriately for the environmental conditions.
5. Keep clients' nails trimmed. Soak the nails before trimming. (*Note:* Know which clients' nails are not to be trimmed by assistants. *Normally, clients with circulatory problems and those who are diabetic have nails trimmed by the professional staff only!*)
6. Guard against pulling the client's skin when assisting with transfers. Skin can tear easily.
7. Avoid drafts within the environment as much as possible.

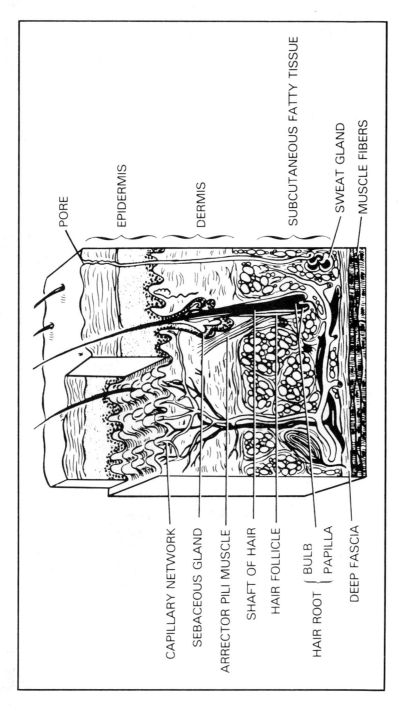

Figure 2.1. Integumentary system: the skin

PORE

EPIDERMIS

DERMIS

SUBCUTANEOUS FATTY TISSUE

SWEAT GLAND

MUSCLE FIBERS

CAPILLARY NETWORK

SEBACEOUS GLAND

ARRECTOR PILI MUSCLE

SHAFT OF HAIR

HAIR FOLLICLE

HAIR ROOT { BULB
{ PAPILLA

DEEP FASCIA

8. Assist the client with exercises and ambulation as much as possible to prevent pressure areas from developing.

9. If clients must be in wheelchairs or are confined to bed, change positions frequently (*every 1 to 2 hours*) to avoid pressure areas. Check the vulnerable skin areas, such as hips, sacral area, and buttocks, each time the client is repositioned.

10. Protect bony prominences from rubbing hard objects, from wrinkled bed linens, and from wrinkled clothing.

11. Involve the client in protecting his or her own skin.

Circulatory System: Heart and Blood Vessels

Heart (Figure 2.2)

Changes	Consequences of Changes
Decrease in cardiac output of blood supply	Sudden illnesses may cause rapid heart rate and inadequate supply of blood and oxygen throughout the body
Fatty deposit accumulation within heart and blood vessels	
Decreased enzyme action on the heart reduces the force and speed of heart contractions	Blood pressure may drop upon sudden change of body position—from lying to walking
Decreased heart rate	Mental confusion may occur
Decreased ability of the heart to return to normal when illness or increased activity occurs	
Tendency for increase in blood pressure	

Blood vessels (Figure 2.3)

Changes	Consequences of Changes
Accumulation of fatty deposits and cholesterol in vessels—arteriosclerosis	Poor circulation to the extremities
Decrease in venous return to the heart, valves in vessels weaken	Feet and hands become cold
	Increase in blood pressure
	Tendency for circulatory disturbances of legs, feet, and hands
	Swelling of lower extremities

Geriatric nursing assistant responses   The following actions can be taken by the geriatric nursing assistant to compensate for changes in the heart and blood vessels that occur in older clients.

1. Provide times of the day for activity and relaxation. Prevent overexertion to avoid stressing the heart.

2. Monitor the lower extremities for edema or swelling. Report any edema present. Elevate the feet above the knee level to reduce swelling when the client is in a sitting position. The nursing care plan should reflect this.

3. Allow clients to change position slowly, especially from a lying position to a sitting position to a standing position, to allow for circulatory changes and adjustment.

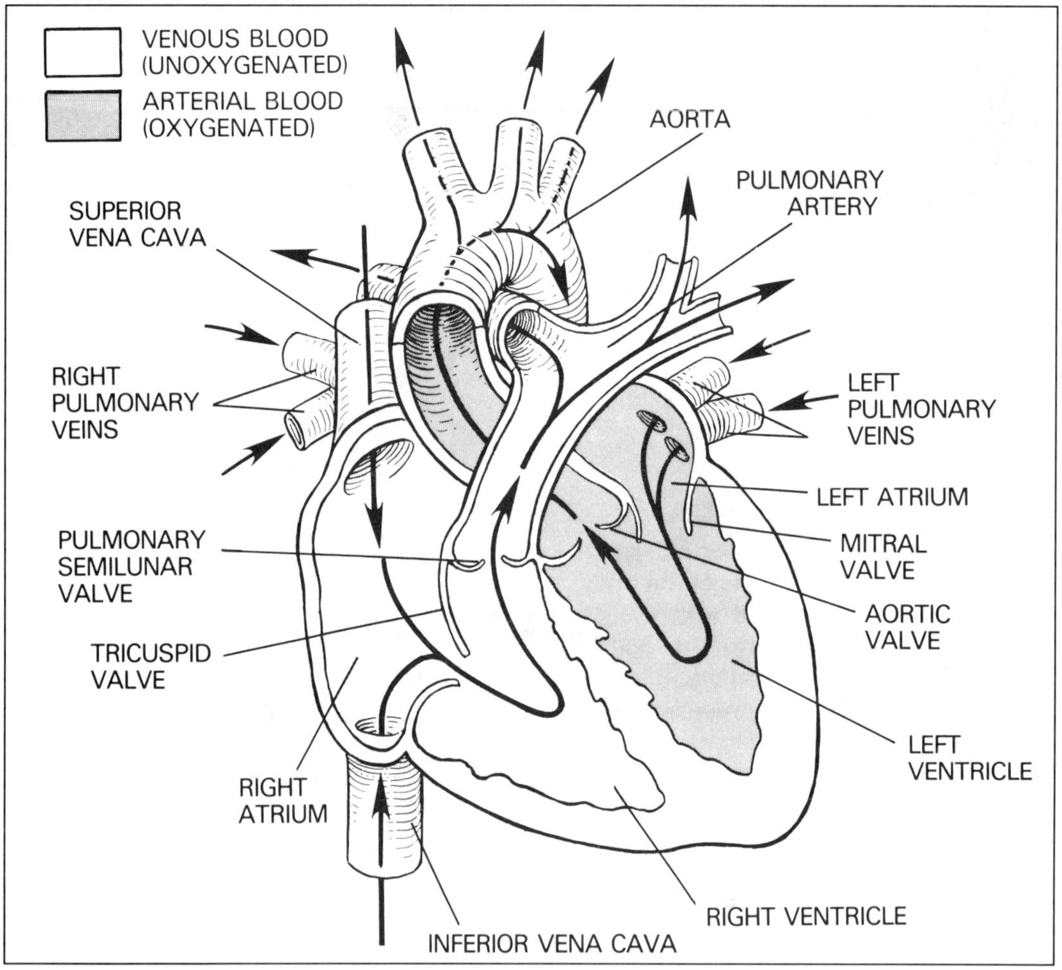

Figure 2.2.   Heart

4. Monitor pulse before, during, and after any unusual increased activity. Know the client's baseline pulse and report any unusual pulse increases, irregularity of beat, and change in volume.

5. Provide foot care and report any unusual appearance: changes in color from normal to blanching (whiteness) to redness. Any complaints of pain in the lower extremities or toes should be reported immediately.

6. Monitor blood pressure readings and report any drastic changes which are much lower or much higher than the normal blood pressure for that client.

7. Provide warm feet and hand coverings as needed for cold hands and feet.

Respiratory System (Figure 2.4)

Changes	*Consequences of Changes*
Lung becomes restricted by rib cage, which calcifies and has less expansion	Dyspnea occurs on exertion
Less oxygen and CO_2 exchanged
Breathing more shallow
Anterior-posterior dimension of the rib cage increases;	Tendency for lower lung bases to collapse

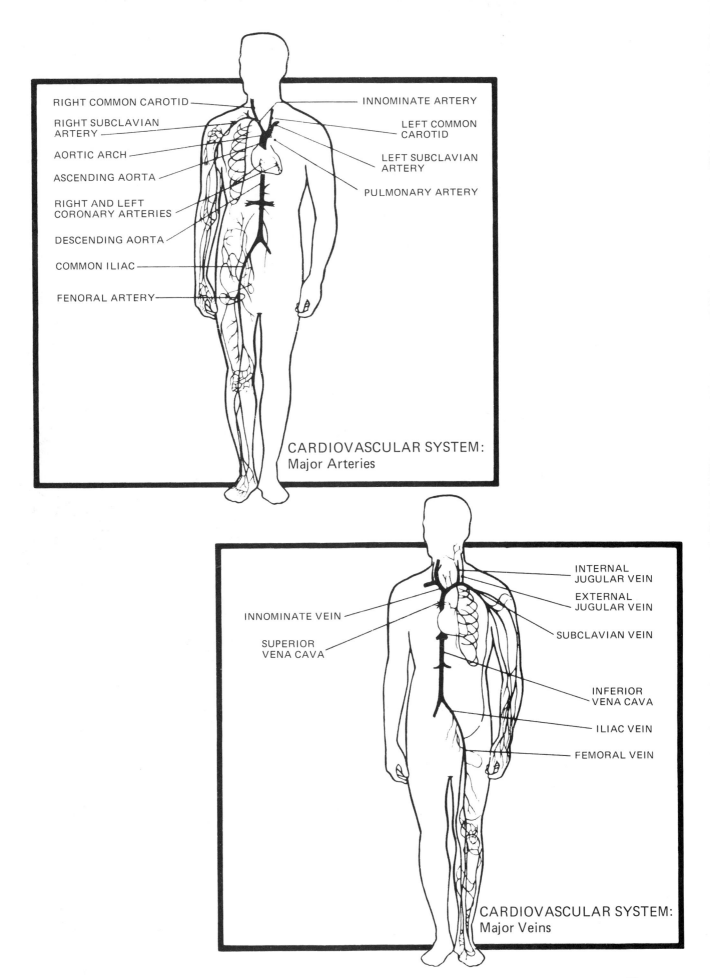

Figure 2.3. Blood vessels

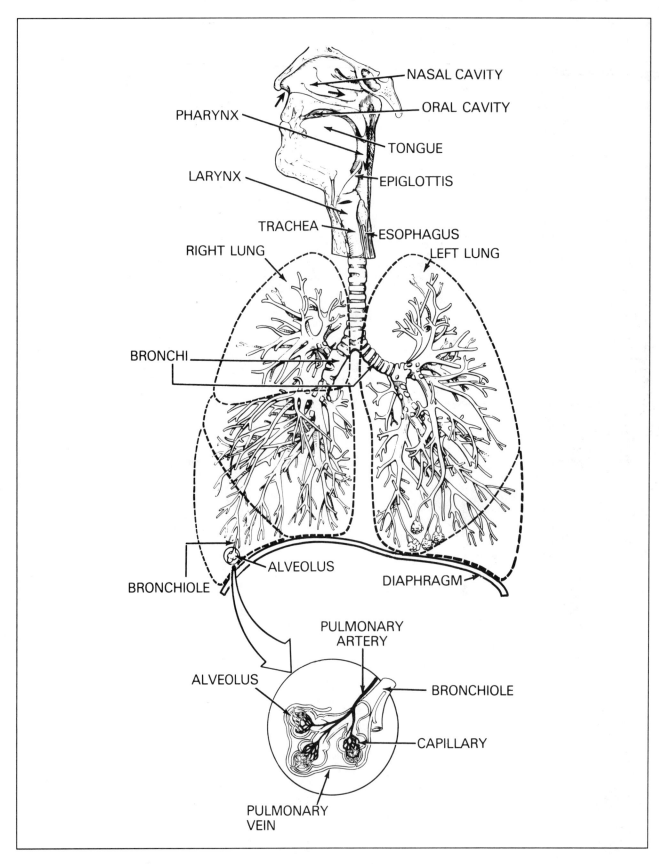

Figure 2.4. Respiratory system

Changes	*Consequences of Changes*
kyphosis may develop (stooped curvature of thoracic spine), but the thoracic transverse dimension decreases	Less effective and productive cough reflex
Lung tissue becomes more rigid	Tendency for lung disease, if inactive
Lungs do not expand fully	
Decreased respiratory muscle strength	
Lower lung tissue at base of the lung expands less; upper lung tissue expands more	

Geriatric nursing assistant responses   The following actions can be taken by the geriatric nursing assistant to compensate for the changes in the respiratory system that occur in older clients.

1. Monitor and report any sudden changes in client's respirations.
2. Slowly assist client in changes of activity to allow time for breathing adjustment without causing fatigue.
3. Have client breathe as deeply as possible routinely throughout the day, 10 deep breaths every hour.
4. Assist clients with physical activities that encourage lung exercise and body mobility.
5. Have clients avoid contact with visitors who have upper respiratory disease, colds, and so on.
6. Encourage postural exercise, which helps to maintain an erect body posture and permits maximum thoracic expansion.

Musculoskeletal System

Muscular system (Figure 2.5)

Changes	*Consequences of Changes*
Decreased number of muscle fibers and muscle tissue	Inactivity results in more loss of strength in lower activities
Muscle strength decreases	Postural changes result in instability of gait
Muscle size decreases and muscles atrophy	Loss of strength tends to produce falls, lessens grip, and reduces ability to perform activities of daily living
Increased waste products are retained in muscle (lactic acid, carbon dioxide)	Muscle cells which are replaced by collagen cause stiffness
Muscle cells accumulate fat and collagen	Accumulated waste products reduce muscle activity

Skeletal system (Figure 2.6)

Changes	*Consequences of Changes*
Bones become porous and brittle	Osteoporosis—occurs more often in women than in men
Bone mass declines	

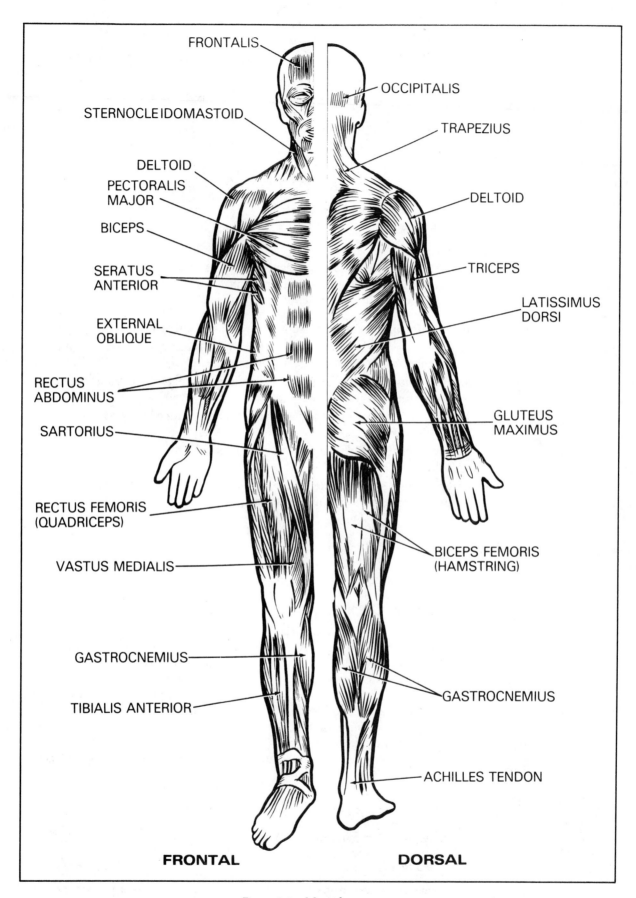

FRONTALIS

OCCIPITALIS

STERNOCLEIDOMASTOID

TRAPEZIUS

DELTOID

PECTORALIS
MAJOR

DELTOID

BICEPS

SERATUS
ANTERIOR

TRICEPS

EXTERNAL
OBLIQUE

LATISSIMUS
DORSI

RECTUS
ABDOMINUS

SARTORIUS

GLUTEUS
MAXIMUS

RECTUS FEMORIS
(QUADRICEPS)

VASTUS MEDIALIS

BICEPS FEMORIS
(HAMSTRING)

GASTROCNEMIUS

TIBIALIS ANTERIOR

GASTROCNEMIUS

ACHILLES TENDON

FRONTAL

DORSAL

Figure 2.5. Muscular system

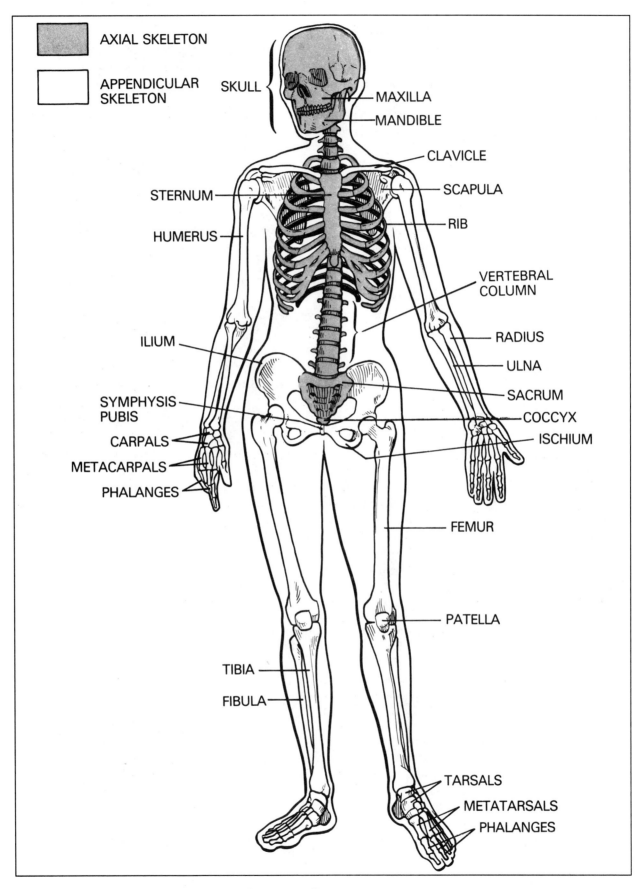

Figure 2.6. Skeletal system

Changes	*Consequences of Changes*
Calcium leaves the bone (especially in women after menopause)	Fractures occur more easily Joints become stiff and mobility is decreased
Curvatures develop in the spine (kyphosis, lordosis)	
Decreased elasticity and ability to move joints	
Joints develop spurs	

Geriatric nursing assistant responses   The following actions can be taken by the geriatric nursing assistant to compensate for musculoskeletal changes that occur in older clients.

1. Assist clients with correct alignment when in bed and to maintain posture when erect.
2. Assist clients, using gentleness, when positioning, transferring, and ambulating.
3. Provide a protective environment which eliminates obstacles, to prevent falls as much as possible. Assure the use of siderails and assistive devices.
4. Encourage nutritional supplements that provide protein and minerals to the client's diet.
5. Increase client's involvement in exercise and activity and in self-care for completion of daily activities.
6. Provide an emotional environment that offers encouragement to do self-care and to improve.
7. Report any noticeable changes that may indicate musculoskeletal involvement: pain, bruises, abnormal distortion of limbs, and sudden restricted movement of limbs.

Digestive System (Figure 2.7)

Changes	*Consequences of Changes*
Loosening of teeth; gum recession	Edentulousness increased (tooth loss)
Loss of tastes; taste buds decreased	False dentures increased Poor appetite
Decrease in enzyme action in all parts of the system	Nutritional deficiencies (protein, vitamins, minerals)
Less hydrochloric acid in the stomach	Increased gum disease Increased food intolerance
Decreased peristalsis and bowel tone	Choking occurs more easily Aspiration possible
Decreased ability to tolerate fat	Constipation increased
Dcreased absorption of vitamins and minerals (vitamins B and K) (calcium and iron)	Less protein intake because of inability to chew meats
Sphincter control of espophagus and large bowel decreased	Tendency for hiatal hernia (A portion of the stomach rises up through the esophageal
Decreased gag reflex	opening of the diaphram.)

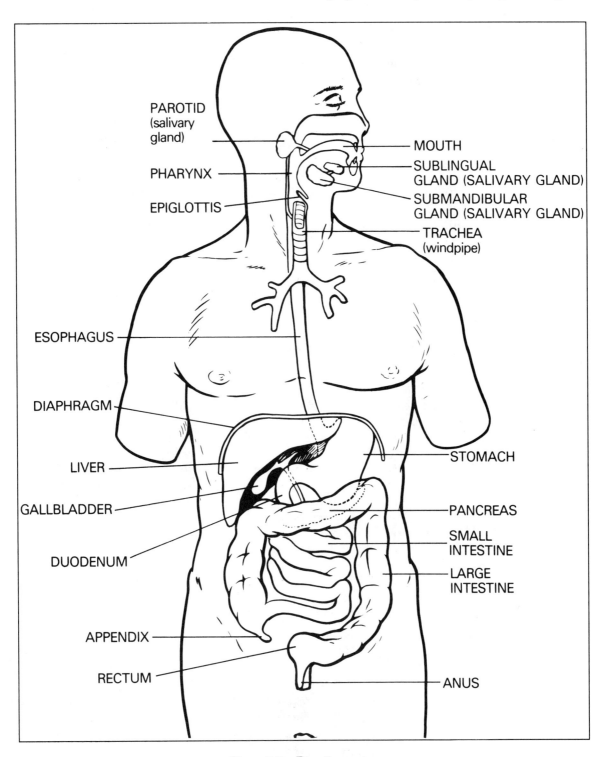

Figure 2.7. Digestive system

Geriatric nursing assistant responses   The following actions can be taken by the geriatric nursing assistant to compensate for digestive system changes that occur in older clients.

1. Assist clients to eat and drink adequate amounts of a balanced diet of solids and liquids.

2. Report the need to change the consistency of foods for easier chewing and swallowing.

3. Assist in making mealtime pleasant.

4. Give clients enough time to chew and swallow.

5. Assist clients to select foods they like.

6. Encourage clients to feed themselves at their own pace.

7. Provide assistive devices as needed (plate guards, utensils with enlarged handles).

8. Provide for supplementary feedings to aid weight gain if needed.

9. Monitor the weight of clients who have poor appetites and show weight loss. Report this to the nurse in charge.

10. Encourage activity to stimulate appetite and bowel activity.

11. Offer prune juice, bran, extra fluids, and fruits to guard against constipation. Report constipation to the nurse in charge.

12. Work with nursing staff to establish a bowel care regime for clients who have a tendency for constipation.

Endocrine (Glandular) System (Figure 2.8)

Changes	Consequences of Changes
Decreasing number of cells and size of glands	Tendency for hypothyroidism
Decreased amounts of secretions from glands	Tendency for diabetes (adult onset)
Decreased basic metabolic rate	Tendency for autoimmune diseases and lowered resistance to disease
Decreased ability to adapt to stress (less adrenalin)	Body temperature decreases; tendency to be cold
Decreased immune response	Females prone to vaginal infections (decreased secretions)
Increased blood glucose levels	
Decreased thyroid secretions	Males: slower ejaculations (decreased secretions)

Geriatric nursing assistant responses   The following actions can be taken by the geriatric nursing assistant to compensate for endocrine system changes that occur in older clients.

1. Provide for an environment free of drafts; protect against a cold environment when assisting client in dressing.

2. Assist clients with daily perineal care to keep them clean and free of infection. Report any signs or symptoms of perineal discomfort.

3. Monitor diabetic clients' eating patterns and report to the nurse in charge any foods not eaten.

4. Encourage exercise and activity to increase blood flow throughout the body.

5. Protect clients from exposure to infectious diseases (staff and visitors with infectious diseases should not come in contact with older clients).

6. Report any new signs or symptoms of possible illnesses to the nurse in charge.

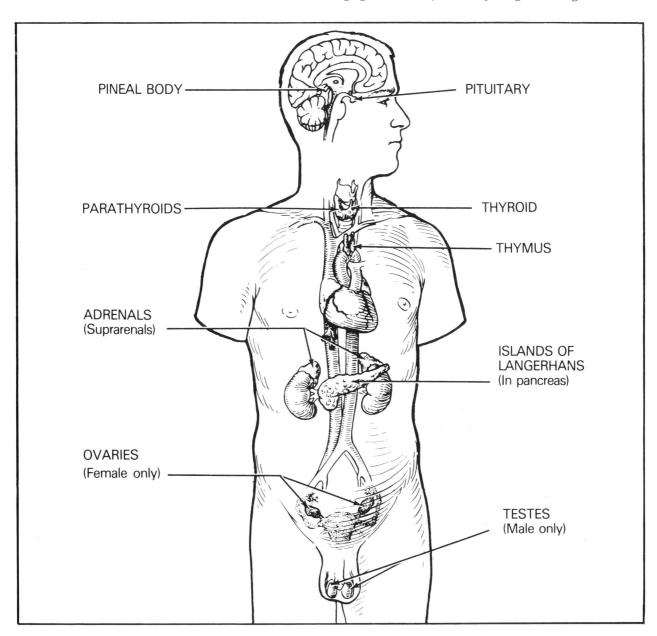

Figure 2.8. Endocrine system

Urinary System (Figure 2.9)

Changes	*Consequences of Changes*
Decrease in size of kidneys	Less ability of kidney to eliminate medications
Decrease in functional cells	
Decrease in vascular circulation to kidneys	Tendency for acid-base imbalance of electrolytes and elimination of body fluids
Less urine produced and excreted	
Reduced filtering function of kidneys	Tendency for nocturnal urination (nocturia) and frequency of urination

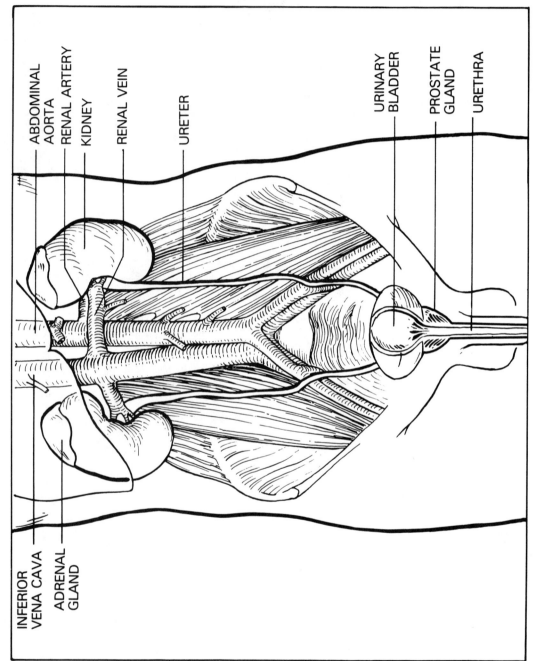

INFERIOR
VENA CAVA

ADRENAL
GLAND

ABDOMINAL
AORTA

RENAL ARTERY

KIDNEY

RENAL VEIN

URETER

URINARY
BLADDER

PROSTATE
GLAND

URETHRA

Figure 2.9. Urinary system

Changes	Consequences of Changes
Decreased muscular tone of pelvic muscles and muscles of urinary bladder	Tendency for urinary infections
	Tendency for urinary retention
	Tendency for incontinence
Decreased ability of bladder to hold urine	Less time between sensation to void and need to void

Geriatric nursing assistant responses   The following actions can be taken by the geriatric nursing assistant to compensate for urinary system changes that occur in older clients.

1. Assure adequate intake of fluids daily—2000 ml per day.
2. Encourage muscle exercises to increase the muscle tone of the bladder (may require help from the physical therapist).
3. Encourage general exercises that improve general circulation to the kidneys and may improve kidney function.
4. Establish a urinary regime with clients who need assistance in getting to the bathroom.
5. Assist the nursing staff in activities that help clients with urinary incontinence.
6. Provide nursing care to prevent skin irritation to clients who cannot be helped with incontinence.
7. Create an environment of encouragement for clients who want to overcome incontinence.

Reproductive System

Female (Figure 2.10A)

Male (Figure 2.10B)

Changes	Consequences of Changes
Females: Decrease in size of ovaries and uterus atrophy occurs; reduced hormonal secretions in vagina; vaginal lining becomes thinner	*Females:* Tendency to experience pruitis (itching) and irritation of vagina; tendency for prolapsed uterus (especially after many pregnancies)
Males: Enlarged prostrate; decrease in size of testes; ejaculations are slowed; sexual function and sexual activity continues for both sexes; more time is required for satisfaction	*Males:* Problems with urination due to obstruction from enlarged prostrate interfering with urine flow

Geriatric nursing assistant responses   The following actions can be taken by the geriatric nursing assistant to compensate for reproductive system changes that occur in older clients.

1. Appreciate the need for love, affection, and expression of both by older men and women.
2. Respect and protect the right of older couples to be alone.
3. Be on the alert for vaginal irritation of female clients. The vaginal tract is subject to irritation; inflammation, and infection. Report any changes.

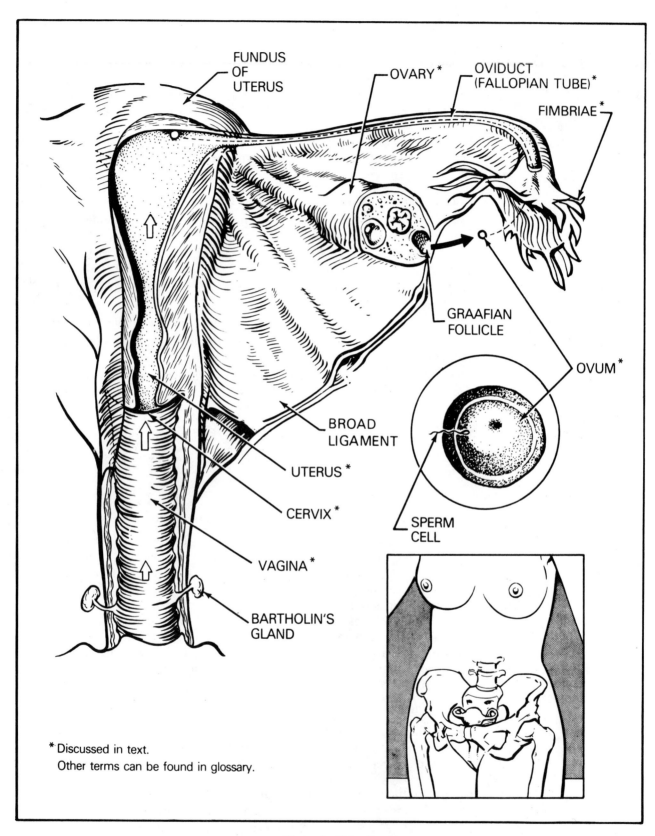

FUNDUS OF UTERUS

OVARY *

OVIDUCT (FALLOPIAN TUBE) *

FIMBRIAE *

GRAAFIAN FOLLICLE

OVUM *

BROAD LIGAMENT

UTERUS *

CERVIX *

SPERM CELL

VAGINA *

BARTHOLIN'S GLAND

* Discussed in text.
Other terms can be found in glossary.

Figure 2.10(a). Female

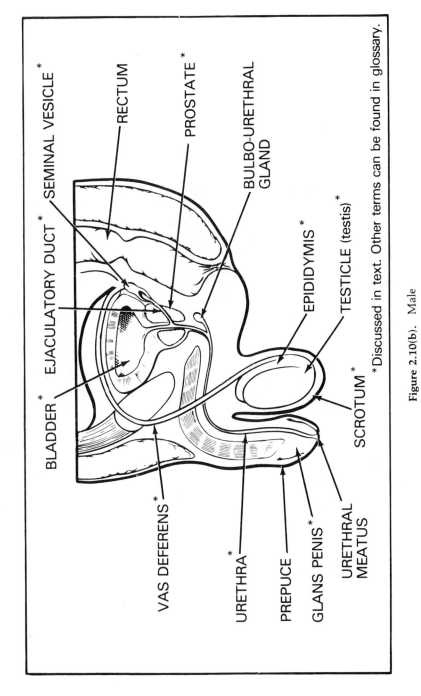

BLADDER *

EJACULATORY DUCT *

SEMINAL VESICLE *

RECTUM

PROSTATE *

BULBO-URETHRAL GLAND

EPIDIDYMIS *

TESTICLE (testis) *

VAS DEFERENS *

URETHRA *

PREPUCE

GLANS PENIS *

URETHRAL MEATUS

SCROTUM *

*Discussed in text. Other terms can be found in glossary.

Figure 2.10(b). Male

4. Report any urinary discomfort and suspected enlargement of the prostrate in males. Surgery may be necessary.
5. Report any suspicion of protrusion of the uterus into the vagina of a female client.

Nervous System (Figure 2.11)

Changes	*Consequences of Changes*
Decrease in brain weight	Activities of daily living take more time
Decrease in neurons (neural cells)	Slower responses to external stimuli
Decrease in psychomotor reaction time as a result of slower conduction time of stimuli to the brain	Learning continues but takes more time
Decrease in blood flow to the brain	Adjustments and devices needed for hearing, vision, and touch
Decrease in all sensory perceptins: hearing, vision, taste, smell, touch, sense of balance	Tendency for falls

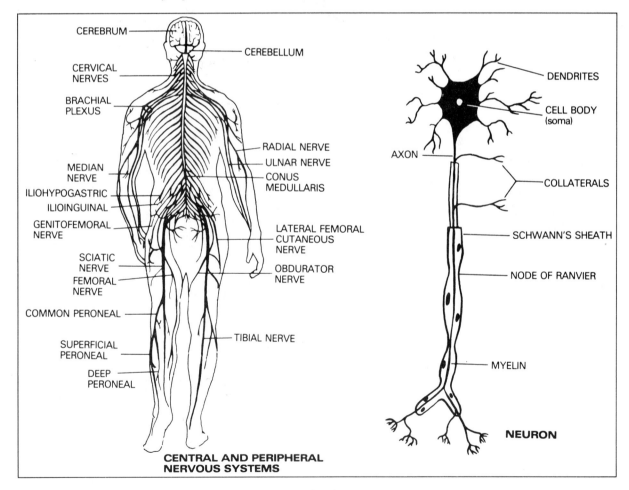

Figure 2.11. Nervous system

Memory may decline
Plaques form within brain tissue

Geriatric nursing assistant responses   The following actions can be taken by the geriatric nursing assistant to compensate for nervous system changes that occur in older clients.

1. Provide time for older adults to respond to directions and change.
2. Assure that clients are using devices needed to improve their sensory perception: eyeglasses, hearing aids, canes, walkers, and braces (and that they are in good working condition).
3. Keep the environment clear of obstacles so that clients can ambulate freely.
4. Provide assistance as needed to help clients exercise and move about without falling.
5. Provide enough light so that clients can see.
6. Follow guidelines when helping hearing impaired clients (see Unit 3).
7. Use reality orientation to help client's memory (see Unit 11).

THE AGING PROCESS: EXPECTED EMOTIONAL AND SOCIAL CHANGES

Emotional Changes

As people grow older, emotional needs do not change, but the ways these needs are met may change. The basic need to be loved and to share affection with a spouse calls for adjustment when the spouse is no longer living. The losses experienced by the older person come in various ways and require a series of adjustments. Emotional reaction to the losses usually reflect the reactions that individuals had to make to adjustments in early life. Many older people who maintain good health, economic independence, and have positive coping mechanisms are able to accept and adjust to changes in their lives. If the person has a chronic illness, little income, and no one to help, the stress encountered may be too severe for the elderly person to live alone. Various emotional reactions may develop, such as fear, loneliness, loss of self-esteem, and depression. As a rule, the more positive the outlook a person has on life's problems, the easier the adjustments are to make as one ages.

Social Changes

As the years go by and we grow and mature, the roles we take on change as well. Some of the roles we have are: child, teenager, student, daughter, son, wife, husband, parent, and grandparent. In the work world we take on such roles as teacher, salesperson, doctor, nurse, chemist, or any work role we choose. As we age, the stage of retirement approaches if we have been part of the work force. Retirement can be a happy, pleasant time when one can enjoy travel and leisure activities and plan new goals. For others, retirement may cause confusion, loss of self-esteem, severe loss of financial support, and withdrawal from social contacts. The elderly person who faces the changes in roles as a natural progression of life, adjusts easily to different circumstances, and finds new ways to meet social changes will find aging a satisfying time. The way the elderly person faced life in earlier years has a great deal to do with his or her life in the advanced years.

THE TOTAL PERSON: NEEDS ASSESSMENT

Approximately 5 percent of those over 65 years of age live in nursing homes. With the expected increase in the aging population, especially elders over 75 years, there will be a proportionate increase in the need for nursing home care. It becomes important for geriatric nursing assistants to be able to help nursing home clients to live a satisfying life. To provide such help, the geriatric nursing assistant participates in defining the needs of each client and contributes to the plan of care.

One way of thinking about needs was developed by Abraham Maslow. Maslow believed that people are motivated to satisfy needs. He established what is known as the hierarchy of needs: Needs have levels, and the basic biological needs must be met first. For example, the infant must be fed and nurtured in order to grow physically and psychologically. The infant's personality develops as these basic needs are satisfied. As the person grows, needs at a higher level serve as a motivating force, and the person is called on to exert energy to meet higher-level needs. The ultimate need is that of self-actualization. Maslow maintained that self-actualization was achieved with maturity and that only the older person becomes self-actualized.

Maslow also believed that self-actualized people have a superior perception of reality and an increased acceptance of self, of other people, and of nature. To achieve the experience of fulfilling one's potential or becoming self-actualized, all other needs have to be satisfied.

A diagram of Maslow's hierarchy of needs is in Figure 2.12. An explanation of each level of need follows.

Biologic integrity. All physiological supports are intact: air, water, food, shelter, sex, comfort. The person is able to satisfy these.

Safety and security. The senses are intact; the environment is safe; there is legal and economic protection; and there is protection from physical, mental, and verbal abuse.

Belonging and love. The person has family, friends, and personal relationships; social integration; affiliations with organizations; and community supports.

Self-esteem and ego satisfaction. The person has control over his or her life; has useful roles; has cultural, spiritual, and psychological supports; is mentally aware; and feels very good about himself and herself.

MASLOW'S HIERARCHY OF NEEDS

Highest level	Self-actualization
	Self-esteem and ego satisfaction
	Belonging and love
	Safety and security
Lowest level	Biologic integrity

Figure 2.12. Maslow's hierarchy of needs.

Self-actualization. The person has reached her/his maximum potential of talents and abilities. Has a legacy to pass on to others.

The needs listed above are integrated, with one need often depending on other needs. The person may place a priority on needs at varying levels, each person being different. The frail elderly person with physical or psychological problems, or both, will have far less energy to meet his or her needs satisfactorily. It then becomes the role of the multidisciplinary team to assess what needs are not being met and to establish a plan of care that will assist the aging person to meet the needs whenever possible. The geriatric nursing assistant is a vital part of the multidisciplinary team.

Another way of defining Maslow's set of needs is to classify them according to the way the needs are generally categorized in nursing: physical, emotional, sociological, cultural, spiritual, and environmental. Figure 2.13 shows that comparison.

The caregiving nursing assistant is in a prime position to look at the total needs of the client and to work with the client in restoring the energy needed to be self-actualized. The purpose of this entire program is to help the specialized nursing assistant to find ways of helping clients become self-actualized. To do this, the nursing assistant must get to know the clients, must know who they are as persons, and must know what they have accomplished in life.

Older people who feel that they accomplished what they wanted to do in life accept themselves and their life's situation with a positive outlook. Some elders do not feel good about themselves because they were not able to satisfy all their needs. The nursing assistant can learn the particular needs of older clients and can work toward helping the other person satisfy them. The care plan of each older person is based on the assessed needs. The plan of care is a product of the problem-solving process. Needs may be called problems because the unsatisfied needs interfere with optimal functioning. The plan of care identifies the problems or needs and the actions to be taken to satisfy the need or to overcome the problem. Let's take as an example a right-handed person who has limited ability to move the right wrist because of joint stiffness due to arthritis (inflammation of the joint). The nursing assistant provides range-of-motion exercises to the person's right wrist. These exercises help the person move the wrist to eat and to perform other functions. Periodically, the physical therapist can evaluate the movements of the person's wrist to be sure that the exercises are helping. If the exercises are not providing enough improvement, the physical therapist may suggest another form of treatment, such as warm packs or more exercises with equipment in the physical therapy department. The physical therapist will consult with

Level	Maslow's Hierarchy	Nursing Categories of Need
I	Biologic integrity	Physical
II	Safety and security	Physical, environmental, emotional
III	Belonging and love	Psychological, sociological, emotional
IV	Ego strength and self-esteem	Psychological, spiritual, cultural, sociological
V	Self-actualization	Social, psychological, spiritual, environmental, cultural, physical, emotional—all needs satisfied

Figure 2.13. Maslow's hierarchy compared to nursing categories of need.

EXAMPLE OF A PLAN OF CARE

Name _____   Diagnosis _____

Problem/Need	Nursing Responses	Evaluation
Stiff right wrist—has difficulty eating; cannot comb hair.	1. R.O.M. to right wrist for 10 min: 9 AM and 3 PM.	1. Slowly increasing movement. Eats with difficulty. 12/30/88 Cannot comb hair with right hand.
	2. To P.T. 11 AM daily for paraffin soak to rt. wrist starting 1/2/89.	2. Can move right wrist freely. Eating and combing hair without difficulty. 1/15/89.

Figure 2.14. Example of a plan of care.

the person's doctor, who will write an order for the additional therapy. The orders will be transferred into nursing actions which will be placed on the plan of care. The nursing staff will know what actions are needed. The additional therapy will then be evaluated for improvement in the motion the person can accomplish with the right wrist (Figure 2.14). It was mentioned in the Preface that the problem-solving process is a continuous process. In this case, the plan of care is a visible, written plan, which tells the nursing assistant what actions or responses are needed. The geriatric nursing assistant helps to evaluate the result of nursing actions and reports what she/he observes to the nurse in charge.

KEY POINTS

1. The theories of aging help us to understand why some changes occur; however, there is no generally accepted theory as to why we age.
2. It is often difficult but necessary to distinguish the processes of aging from hidden infections or disease processes. Residents have been labeled "senile" when confusion occurs because of an undiagnosed condition that is treatable.
3. Experience has proven that it is the satisfaction of psychological needs, spiritual needs, or other dimensions of human needs which have helped many elderly improve in health.
4. Encourage the use of the resident's energy to promote self-care and optimal functioning. Involve the resident in his or her own care.
5. Allow for decisions to be made by the resident whenever possible.
6. Recognize that the older person has had many emotional and social changes in a lifetime. Each change requires an adjustment.
7. The older person within a nursing home has usually suffered several losses.
8. Identifying and meeting the needs of older clients is a continuous problem-solving process. The plan of care is a visible, written product that is based on problem solving and need identification. It is a product that must change as needs/problems change.

SELF-CHECK

1. Theories of aging try to explain why people age.
   a. The theory that relates to the elder person's inability to resist disease is called _____ .
   b. The theory which states that aging is caused by pieces of molecules breaking off to attach to other molecules is called _____ .
   c. The theory which states that we have a specific time to die and that death is controlled by the genes is called _____ .
2. List the body systems, with three age-related changes, and then list as many nursing assistant responses as you can for each of the system changes.

3. List the five levels of need defined by Abraham Maslow.

4. What would keep an 80-year-old widower with deafness and chronic heart disease from satisfying his needs? (Use the problem-solving approach in thinking about your answers.)

5. Mrs. Smith is a 70-year-old widow who lives alone on Social Security income. She owns her own home, drives her own car, and volunteers at the local elementary school. She was a schoolteacher before she retired. What emotional and social changes have probably occurred in her life?

SUGGESTED ACTIVITIES

1. Talk with an elderly family member or friend of the family about the physical, emotional, and social changes that have occurred in his or her lifetime and what adjustments had to be made.
2. Visit a senior citizens' center and talk with the elderly people there about their lifestyles and how they view aging.
3. Investigate the activities available for the elderly and find out how many people take advantage of them.
4. Ask your instructor about inviting some elderly people to your class to discuss how they meet their needs.

5. Look at Maslow's hierarchy of needs and be able to discuss how you meet your own needs.

CLINICAL APPLICATION

Using the problem-solving worksheet provided, select from among the elderly persons for whom you give care a client who communicates well. Talk with the client to obtain information that is not available from the care plan and chart. Use the problem-solving process to guide your responses. Complete the assessment and provide geriatric nursing assistant responses to help the person meet his or her needs for optional functioning. When the worksheet is completed, turn it in to your instructor.

WORKSHEET

Interpretation of a Client's Needs and Meeting Those Needs through Nursing Responses

Basic biologic integrity. Are body systems functioning without problems? Respiration, circulation, nutrition, elimination, skin integrity, sleep, rest, exercise, activities, comfort, sexuality. Are there any problems with breathing, blood circulation, skin breakdown, and so on? Example of a problem: Has constipation, severe at times.

Problems: (List briefly)

Nursing responses currently given to meet problems: (List briefly)

Suggestions for improvement:

Safety and security. Consider if all senses are intact: Is the person blind or hard of hearing? Does the person have a false limb? Are restraints needed? Does the person feel safe? Environmental safety: Is there enough space for mobility? Are rights protected? Example of a problem: Tries to climb over bed rails, falls easily.

Problems: (List briefly)

Nursing responses currently given to meet problems: (List briefly)

Suggestions for improvement:

Belonging and love. Consider if there is communication and interpersonal relationships with friends, family, and care givers. Are there community contacts? Is there expression of sexuality? Example of a problem: No family in the state where the client lives.

Problems: (List briefly)

Nursing responses currently given to meet problems: (List briefly)

Suggestions for improvement:

Ego strength and self-esteem. Consider if he or she copes with daily situations, is mentally alert, maintains control over decisions, makes choices. Does he or she have an opportunity to express wishes to participate in cultural and spiritual preferences? Example of a problem: Will not participate in any activities; is withdrawn.

Problems: (List briefly)

Nursing responses currently given to meet problems: (List briefly)

Suggestions for improvement:

Self-actualization. Uses creativity in daily or frequent experiences; has a legacy to leave to the world; is able to see meaning and purpose in life; accepts death as an eventuality; participates in leisure and recreational activity; has a pattern of daily life that reflects peace and happiness; has a feeling of mastery over daily life. Example of a problem: Calls out in fear or expresses unhappiness over being in the nursing home.

Problems: (List briefly)

Nursing responses currently given to meet problems: (List briefly)

Suggestions for improvement:

3 SENSORY LOSSES OF AGING PEOPLE

TERMINAL PERFORMANCE OBJECTIVE

Using a problem-solving approach, be able to provide nursing responses to a client with sensory loss that will assist the client to improve functioning.

Enabling Objectives

1. Identify three conditions commonly found in aging clients that contribute to visual loss and nursing responses which will help the client compensate for these losses.
2. Describe the expected changes in the ear that contribute to a loss in hearing in the aged person.
3. Identify the most common type of hearing loss and nursing measures that can be applied to help the person compensate for the loss.
4. Describe the common changes in taste and smell expected with aging and ways to help the aging person compensate for these losses.
5. Explain why elderly people have less sensitivity to temperature.
6. Describe two conditions that can develop because of insensitivity to temperature changes and the nursing responses to help compensate.
7. Explain changes in the elderly that lead to decreased sensation in the extremities, especially fingers and toes, and the safety measures and nursing responses that are indicated.
8. Select an elderly client with sensory loss; using a problem-solving approach, provide nursing assisting responses and evaluate the outcomes.

REVIEW SECTION

The topics you should review with your instructor are the anatomy and physiology of the eye (Figure 3.1a), ear (Figure 3.1b), nose (Figure 3.1c), and tongue (Figure 3.1d). Also review the changes in the nervous and circulatory systems that contribute to insensitivity to temperature and loss of sensation in the extremities.

IMPACT OF SENSORY LOSSES

Sensory changes in the elderly can result in a loss of function and decrease in the activities of daily living. When compensatory measures are provided, the aging process does not have to cause less independence and decreased functioning. Too frequently a person's changes in the sensorium result in a label of "senile" or "confused." Instead, the care giver should be patient and understanding and provide compensatory changes in the environment to revive the person's functioning abilities. In this unit we provide a review of the major changes in vision, hearing, taste, smell, temperature control, and extremities with compensating measures that can be provided by the geriatric nursing assistant.

SENSORY LOSSES AND TECHNIQUES FOR COMPENSATING*

Changes in Vision

Changes	*Compensations*
1. As a person ages, the lens in the eye yellows and thickens. The muscles that control pupil size also weaken. As a result, the older eye requires more light than the young eye. A 65-year-old eye needs more than twice as much light as does a 20-year-old eye (Figure 3.3).	Provide adequate lighting (Figure 3.2). Be aware of poor lighting and the fact that the older person may be unable to see obstacles, read signs, or recognize familiar people when the lighting is poor. The older person can avoid situations that will call for good vision if the lighting will not be good. For example, many older people will avoid driving at night. Offer to assist an older person who is walking or carrying on an activity when the light is poor.
2. The lens grows unevenly and becomes striated. The lens tends to refract the light that passes through it and causes a glare problem. A small amount of glare that hardly bothers a younger person may cause great difficulties for an older person	Avoid glare from windows by careful adjustment of shades or drapes throughout the day. Avoid shiny surfaces that reflect light. Tabletops, waxed floors, vinyl upholstery materials, and mirrors may create glare. Sunglasses, large-brimmed hats,

*Adapted with permission from the Ebenezer Center for Aging and Human Development, Minneapolis, MN, *Compensating for Sensory Loss*, Kathy Carroll, Ed., 1978, p. 242.

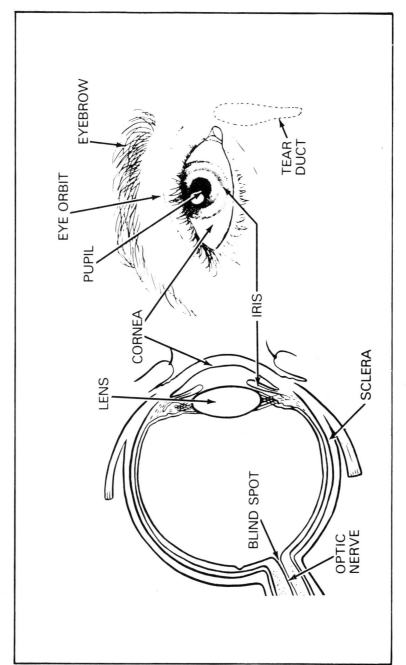

Figure 3.1(a). The eye.

49

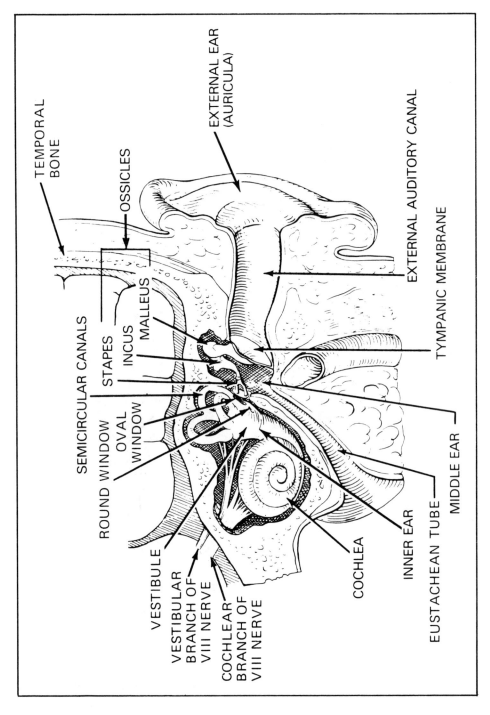

TEMPORAL BONE

OSSICLES

EXTERNAL EAR (AURICULA)

EXTERNAL AUDITORY CANAL

SEMICIRCULAR CANALS

STAPES

INCUS

MALLEUS

TYMPANIC MEMBRANE

ROUND WINDOW

OVAL WINDOW

VESTIBULE

VESTIBULAR BRANCH OF VIII NERVE

COCHLEAR BRANCH OF VIII NERVE

COCHLEA

INNER EAR

EUSTACHEAN TUBE

MIDDLE EAR

Figure 3.1(b). Cross section of the ear.

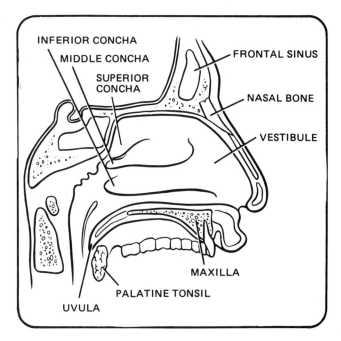

Figure 3.1(c).   The nose.

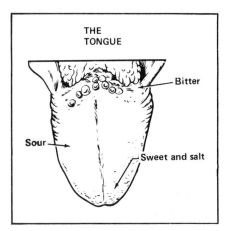

Figure 3.1(d).   The tongue.

Changes	*Compensations*
who is trying to see something. The glare may also cause anxiety and an inability to concentrate.	or sunshades may help when people are outdoors or riding in a car. When people cannot express themselves, staff must be aware of glare problems and watch for signs of anxiety due to glare.
3. Changes in the lens make color perception more difficult. Pastel colors (pink, yellow, pale blue) may all look alike. Brown, dark blue, and black may be difficult to identify correctly.	Do not interpret an inability to identify colors as a sign of confusion. Do not expect older people to use pastels and very dark colors for a color-coding system for example, they should not depend on color to help them take the correct pill.

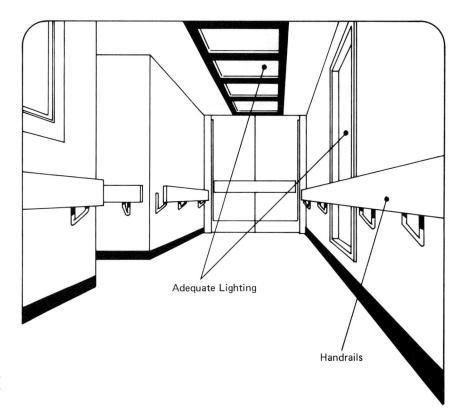

Adequate Lighting

Handrails

Figure 3.2 Handrails and well-lighted corridors assist the visually impaired.

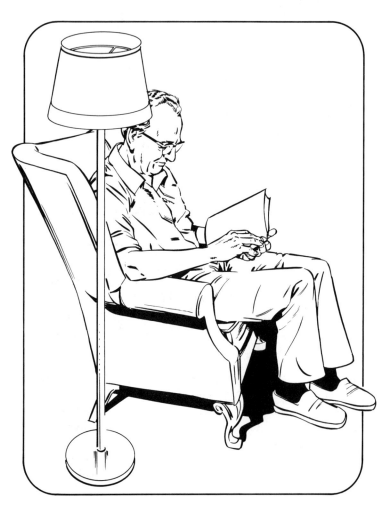

Figure 3.3. Older people need twice as much light as younger people.

Changes	*Compensations*
4. The older eye does not adapt quickly to changes in light level. Abrupt changes in light level can be hazardous and cause falls and other accidents.	Place lights strategically and keep some lights on so that changes in lighting will be more gradual. For example, night lights in bedrooms or a consistent light level in both bedrooms and hallways will help. When there is an abrupt change in the light level, an older person should wait until the eyes have adapted before continuing to walk. Use of handrails can be especially important when there is a change in lighting. If accompanied, an older person should be encouraged to take someone's arm to be guided. Be careful when placing furniture just inside an entryway (Figure 3.4). People who enter a building may bump into things that are just inside the door if their eyes have not yet adjusted to the change in lighting.
5. Conditions of the eye that cause visual loss are very common among older people, so many people have poor visual acuity in their later years. However, most of these people are not totally blind (without light perception) and they can be helped to use their residual vision. Over half of the severe visual impairments occur in people 65 and over. Legal blindness is most common in this age group, too.	Older people should have their eyes examined by an ophthalmologist regularly to assure prevention of eye disease. Acuity information should be provided to the older person. Going closer to things is one of the best ways to see them better. Older people should know that going very close to a TV set will not damage their vision. People who say they are "saving their eyes" by limiting reading and other activity should be told that using their eyes is beneficial and will not hurt them. Things that are extra large are easier to see. This includes large print, dials, controls, and buttons (Figure 3.5). The use of a magnifying glass helps. Contrasting colors make things easier to see. For example, doorways can contrast with the wall, dishes can contrast with the tablecloth (Figure 3.6), the chair seat can contrast with the floor, and personal items can contrast with a covering on the

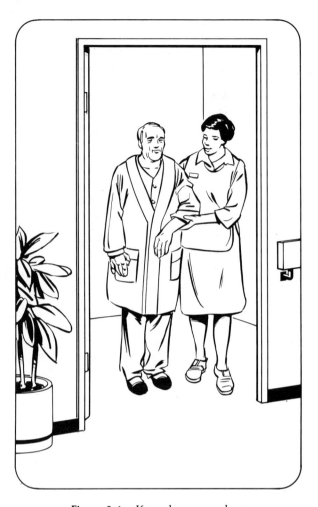

Figure 3.4.   Keep doorways clear.

Changes	*Compensations*
	dresser top. Avoid clutter (Figure 3.7). It is easier to see things with some space between them than when many things are crowded together. Do not change furniture arrangements unless it is necessary to do so; if you do, tell people about it and be sure that they become familiar with the new layout.
6. The changes in vision occur slowly over time and older people are often not aware of them. Sometimes they think that reduced visual acuity is something they should accept as they age and consequently, do not seek help.	Some conditions can be prevented, controlled, or corrected, and older people should be encouraged to see an ophthalmologist regularly to find out whether their vision can be improved.

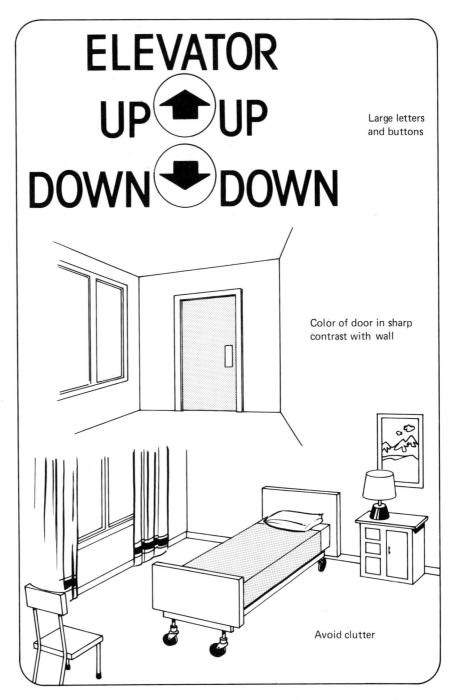

Figure 3.5. Large letters and buttons assist the visually impaired.

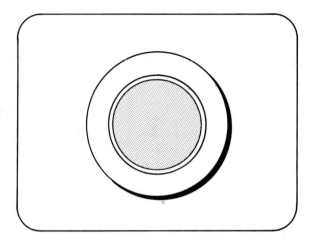

Figure 3.6. Plates in contrast with tablecloth.

Changes	*Compensations*
7. Older persons are most often those who experience cataracts, glaucoma, and macular degeneration.	Older people and their families should be aware of eye diseases, the potential for diagnosis and treatment, and the type of visual deficits that are caused.
8. Glaucoma is an insidious eye disease that has no noticeable symptoms until irreversible damage is done. It involves a loss of vision due to raised intraocular pressure, which damages the optic nerve. Glaucoma can be controlled and vision loss prevented if it is detected in time.	There currently is a simple and painless test for glaucoma and people can be made aware of this and the importance of having the test.

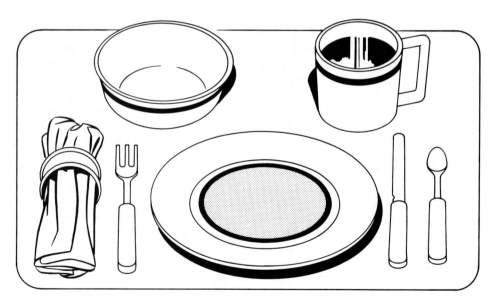

Figure 3.7. Avoid crowding things together. Keep space between utensils.

Changes

9. At this time there is no known prevention for cataracts, but they can be treated successfully by surgical removal of the lens, which has become cloudy and opaque. The surgery is usually not done until the vision loss has become severe. The lack of a natural lens in the eye is compensated by special optical lenses, which can be recognized by their thickness and the magnification of the person's eyes behind them. Cataract glasses make objects seem larger than they really are. It is sometimes very difficult for an older person to adjust to these distortions. A person wearing cataract glasses also has a blind spot at each side where the glasses cannot provide correction. This causes things to appear to pop suddenly into a person's visual field. There is a technique of implanting a lens in the eye at the time of surgery, and this has been very successful. With implanted lenses some of the problems of visual field change and size distortions are solved.

10. Macular degeneration is a condition that causes loss of the central vision as the macula, the area of the retina responsible for central vision, deteriorates. This condition is not preventable or curable. However, as peripheral vision is not affected by the disease, people can be reassured that this will not cause total blindness. There is currently a method being tried to limit the progress of macular degeneration. A laser is used to cauterize the hemorrhaging blood vessels in the retina.

11. There is some indication that there is a relationship between visual loss and mental function.

Compensations

Even if a person has had cataract surgery and wears special cataract glasses, they may still experience some difficulty in seeing. They may need some help reading, crossing the street, and doing other things that we assume should be easy. Try to be aware of these potential needs. People wearing the special lenses may also be unsure of themselves and want what seems to be extra, even unnecessary reassurance or assistance. On the other hand, people who are very proud may need extra assistance but refuse to ask for it. It might help such people to ask how they might be assisted. Some people are self-conscious about the fact that the lenses make their eyes appear to be large and need reassurance about this. To avoid startling someone who wears cataract glasses, approach slowly from the front rather than the side.

Low-vision aids such as magnifying glasses can be of some help to people who are not in the most advanced stage of macular degeneration. People with macular degeneration may not seem to have a severe vision problem. Due to their peripheral vision, they can move around independently without bumping into things and may appear to see quite see quite well. When they talk about their vision problems, some people do not believe them and think they are looking for extra help or attention.

Compensation and correction for vision problems may possibly lead to better mental functioning. It's worth a try!

Changes

12. People who have visual deficits are not able to benefit from the nonverbal feedback that is important when we communicate. They cannot see the smiles, frowns, and other facial expressions that are an important part of conversation.

13. Dining can present special problems for visually impaired people. There may be difficulties in eating independently. Some people are afraid to dine socially because they might spill or make mistakes. Food that is difficult to see is not appealing.

14. People who have vision problems may be unsure of themselves in social situations and

Compensations

When conversing with people who have vision problems, touch can be used to compensate. Holding, squeezing, or patting someone's hand, for example, can tell a person that you are listening and paying attention (Figure 3.8). If people are totally blind, touching them will let them know where you are and assure them that you have not walked away without their being aware of it.

For the people who have low vision, place settings should be uncluttered and make use of contrasting colors while limiting glare. A tablecloth or placemat can help with the glare problem. Someone should name the foods and tell where each is located (Figure 3.9). Finger foods and beverages can be used at snack time to allow people to feel more comfortable about their ability to eat appropriately (Figure 3.10). Blind people may work with an occupational therapist to improve their eating abilities.

Help visually impaired people to look attractive and reassure them honestly about their appear-

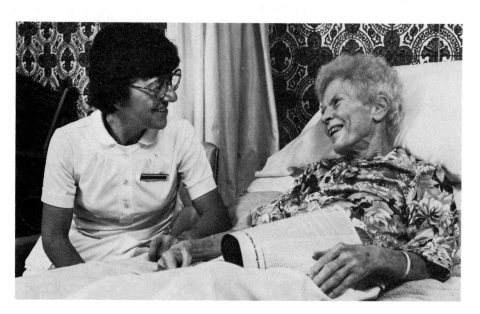

Figure 3.8. Use touch to communicate.

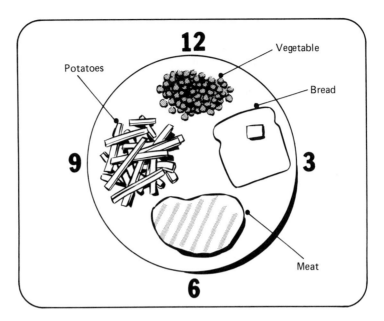

Figure 3.9. Use the clock method to help the visually impaired locate food on the plate.

Changes

may even be fearful if they are in unfamiliar surroundings and situations.

Compensations

ances. Always explain the layout of a room, the people who are there, and where those people are when accompanying them to a social activity. Do not leave them alone until they have someone they can talk with or until they are in contact with a table, chair, or wall that will help with orientation.

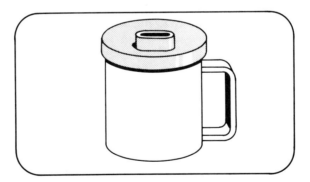

Figure 3.10. Cups with seals help the visually impaired to drink without spilling.

Changes in Hearing

Changes

1. There is a decline in auditory acuity with age called presbycusis. This age-related hearing loss

Compensation

Be aware of the fact that any older person may need your help in compensating for hearing loss.

Changes

is usually greater for men than for women. The reason for this is not known, but is suspected that men are exposed to more damaging noise during their lifetime, in the military service or in their jobs.

2. Loudness is measured in decibels. The decibel, named after Alexander Graham Bell, is the smallest difference in loudness that the human ear can detect. The following list will help to clarify the relationship of decibels to loudness:

Normal breathing	10 decibels
Whisper	30 decibels
Normal speech	60 decibels
Busy traffic	70 decibels
Jet takeoff (discomfort)	140 decibels

3. Hearing loss is worse for high frequencies. This means that some sounds will be heard, whereas others will not. Sounds may be distorted, heard incorrectly, and misinterpreted.

4. People with normal hearing have a wide range between the quietest sound they can hear and loudness that will be painful or irritating. For the hard of hearing this range may be much smaller. Sounds may have to be quite loud to be heard, but if they are even a little louder they

Compensations

While a visually impaired person can compensate by bringing things closer, people with hearing losses cannot compensate themselves; they must depend on others to speak so that they can hear. *Speak slowly and clearly, do not change the topic abruptly. Be sure to face the person at eye level and have light on your face so that lip reading is possible. Ask the person what you can do to make hearing easier.*

Prolonged exposure to 70 decibels or louder can cause hearing loss. Even if people are already hard of hearing, they should conserve the hearing that does remain and avoid exposure to damaging sound.

Try to lower your voice rather than allowing your voice to become high and shrill. Women should be especially careful about this. When a sound system is being used for music, entertainment, or an oral presentation of any kind, it should be adjusted so that the base and lower tones are predominant (Figure 3.11). This will make it easier for hard-of-hearing people to enjoy the music or understand what is being said.

Talk to hard-of-hearing people to find out the very best tone to use with them. Do not assume that simply making things louder will solve the problem. Be aware of the fact that noise or music may be irritating and may cause anxiety for people who are hard of hearing even if it sounds good

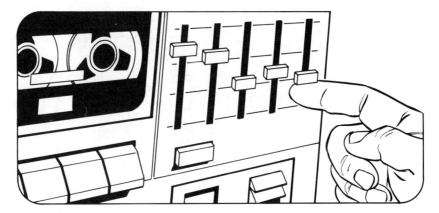

Figure 3.11. Adjust the sound system so base and lower tones are dominant.

Changes	*Compensations*
may be "too loud" to be understood or they may be painful.	*to you. Be especially aware of this when you are working with people who are unable to communicate their needs to you. Note signs of anxiety and try changing noise level.*
5. Hearing loss is greater for consonants than for vowels. "S", "Z", "T", "F", and "G" are particularly difficult to discriminate, causing difficulty in hearing words correctly. Similar words, such as *cat* and *sat*, can be particularly difficult to discriminate.	People should be aware of the fact that even if the sounds can be heard, they may not always be heard correctly. The suggestions mentioned previously can be followed, and in addition, it is helpful to limit the competing stimuli of background noise. Choose a quiet, private place for conversations.
6. Some hearing deficits can be helped by the use of hearing aids. They must be worn and adjusted correctly in order to help. They also require new batteries often. Some people never learn to use their hearing aids correctly or do not get new batteries often enough.	Older people who get hearing aids should be sure to get them from reputable firms and should be trained in their proper use. Family members or staff members of institutions serving older people should also learn about the function and use of hearing aids so that they can help adjust or insert the aid or change batteries if necessary (Figure 3.12). The cost of batteries should be kept in mind. Some people who are concerned with their finances may choose to limit the use of their hearing aids to save on the cost of batteries.

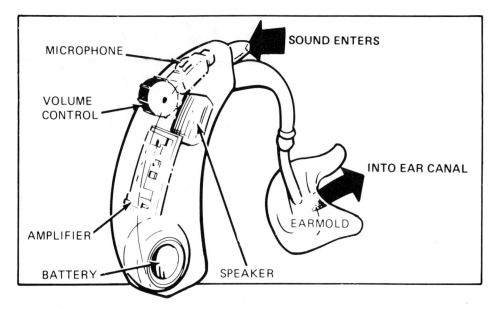

Figure 3.12.   Earmold enlarged to show internal parts.

Changes	*Compensations*
7. Some hearing deficits cannot be helped by hearing aids and the hearing is so poor that verbal communication is difficult.	*Encourage the use of nonverbal communication such as big smiles, waving, pointing, or demonstrating.* Provide items that can be seen and handled as conversation starters. Animals help people to satisfy the need to communicate and to feel loved (Figure 3.13). Offer opportunities for activity and social interaction that do not require spoken communication. For example, cooking and cleaning-up activities can be done by two or more people with good understanding and cooperation in complete silence. Bowling or dancing are other examples. *Do not overlook the potential for writing to communicate.* Even people who appear to be very impaired may be able to understand simple statements and questions that are presented in writing. Large print may be used with those who have vision problems (Figure 3.14).
8. Hearing and following a conversation can take tremendous amounts of effort and energy for a hard-of-hearing person. Moti-	We should try to be more tolerant of "selective hearing." This often annoys people who interact with hard-of-hearing people, but

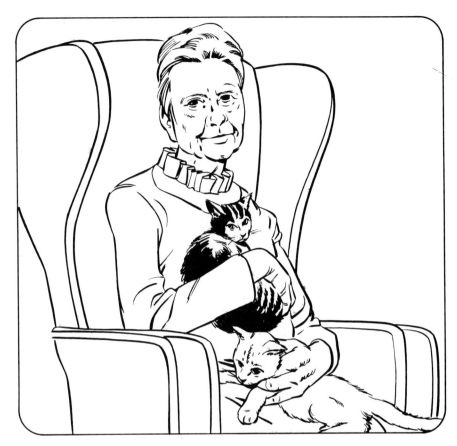

Figure 3.13. Pets serve many useful purposes for the elderly and aid communication.

Changes	*Compensations*
vation, the context of the environment, and general feelings of well-being and energy can make a difference in the ability to understand verbal communication. Lack of any or all of these may result in apparent "selective hearing."	in some cases there may be legitimate reasons for this to occur. Provide opportunities for people to participate in activities that are enjoyable but require little conversation. Playing cards, doing puzzles, preparing food, and taking walks are examples.
9. Depression and paranoid reactions are common among older people with hearing loss. When people cannot hear what is being said, they may begin to think that people are talking about them and saying negative things.	*Do everything possible to compensate for hearing loss and be sure that hard-of-hearing people know what is going on and what the conversation is about. If there is a conversation that does not concern the hard-of-hearing person, tell him/her the topic that is being discussed so that he/she will not feel left out or talked about.*

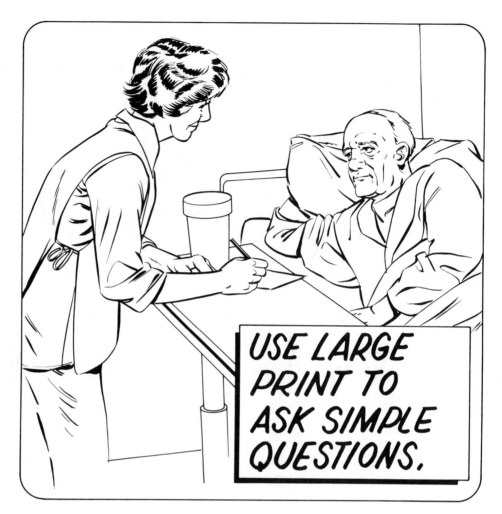

USE LARGE PRINT TO ASK SIMPLE QUESTIONS.

Figure 3.14. Large letters.

Changes	*Compensations*
10. Hearing is important to more than communication. It is also a way of getting signals from the environment and therefore relates to safety.	People who work or live with a hard-of-hearing person should keep this in mind. People in the community should also consider when they see an older person crossing the street that a car or horn may not be heard.

Changes in the Ability to Taste and Smell

Changes	*Compensations*
1. There is an indication that senses of taste and smell decline significantly with age. Elderly people do not perform as well as young people on tasks involving the identification of odors and taste of food. In one recent study, the	Older people probably rely on the appearance of the food for identification and inspiration to eat. People with poor vision may be very limited in their ability to identify foods, causing foods to have little appeal. Dis-

Changes	*Compensations*
foods most often identified by taste and smell were: salt, 89 percent; coffee, 71 percent; tomato, 69 percent; fish, 59 percent; and sugar, 57 percent (Schiffman, 1976).	tinctive textures and temperatures can be important for the and enjoyment of food. Ice cream and popcorn are two popular items in some nursing homes, for example.
2. Poor nutrition can have serious consequences for elderly people, so it is important that they eat properly. Tasteless foods make eating less enjoyable. Bland, low salt, and other diet restrictions can contribute to the undesirability of food.	A pleasant mealtime atmosphere and foods that are enjoyed in a social setting can make people feel more like eating. Talking about the food—the good taste and smell—can make the food appear to taste better. Condiments and foods with strong flavors may also help to maintain interest in food and eating.
3. Poor sense of smell and taste may make it difficult to recognize spoiled foods or the smell of things such as gas. This is a potential hazard for the person who lives alone.	Older people living alone should be encouraged to take this into consideration. They can keep track of the age of foods in their refrigerators and check the pilot lights of gas stoves regularly. Families and friends can also check these things whenever they visit.

Changes in Temperature Control

The loss of sensitivity to temperature becomes a complex situation because of the many body systems that can contribute to the problem. Generally, the age-related changes in distribution of body fat result in a loss of insulation from the skin surfaces. The elderly person chills more frequently. In addition, the muscle tissue that allows a person to shiver and raise body temperature is reduced in the elderly person. The effects of some drugs and alcohol result in depressed stimulation to the temperature control center in the brain.

Elderly people may suffer from confusion brought on by drugs or alcohol and remain in environments that are cold and unhealthy. The presence of a disease that limits mobility, such as arthritis or stroke, and a disease that compounds decreased temperature, such as congestive heart failure, contributes to the loss of body heat. The condition that results from low body temperature is called *hypothermia*. It is defined as a body temperature below 35° C (95°F).

Another condition, *hyperthermia*, results when a person's body heat is greater than 40.6 °C (105 °F). A person who has an altered mental state with a temperature of 40.6 °C (105 °F), is considered to have hyperthermia. Hyperthermia is often diagnosed during severe heat waves in the summer. If the body temperature is not reduced, permanent damage or death occurs.

Although these conditions are not likely to occur in controlled environments such as nursing homes, the geriatric nursing assistant should be aware of them and know how to respond in case he or she suspects that either condition could be developing.

Geriatric nursing assistant responses

1. Check to see that clients are well dressed for the season; some clients will require outer garments even in the summer.
2. Encourage as much exercise as possible to maintain body functions that produce energy and heat when needed.
3. Check on elderly people you know who live alone to see if their home heat is functioning and adequate. Hypothermia can develop with the elderly in this kind of situation, especially when the heat is turned down to save on cost. Symptoms to watch for are: very slow pulse, confusion, low blood pressure, and cold skin. Report any suspicion of hypothermia to responsible and concerned parties. If untreated, hypothermia can result in death.
4. A person with hypothermia requires a slow warming process under a physician's orders. Do not attempt rapid warming measures.
5. A person with hyperthermia requires rapid cooling measures under the direction of a physician. Do attempt to remove a person from an environment of excessive heat. The elderly person should not be exposed to weather that is very hot and humid. Symptoms to watch for are: hot skin with increased perspiration, skin that appears flushed with cyanosis, increased body temperature, disorientation, or confusion—heat stroke is possible. Report any suspicion of hyperthermia to responsible and concerned parties.

Sensory Changes in the Extremities

Some older people have a decreased sensation in the fingers and toes which makes it difficult to tell hot from cold. This diminished sensation can result in burns of the tissue in the hands and feet if the person touches or steps into water and other substances that are hot. The loss of sensation in the extremities especially affects long-term diabetic patients with severe circulatory problems. The geriatric nursing assistant should ask older clients about their ability to feel hot and cold temperatures with their fingers and toes.

KEY POINTS

1. Sensory losses should not interfere with the client's ability to improve and participate in activities of daily living (ADL).
2. Sensory loss in hearing and vision can cause caregivers to label the elderly as senile or confused. Compensating for the loss can restore functioning.
3. A thorough assessment of the client's sensorium, and nursing responses provided to compensate for losses experienced by the client, may make the client's life in the nursing home or elsewhere a very happy one.

SELF-CHECK

1. Mrs. Jones is 90 years old. She complains that even her glasses do not help her with reading the newspaper. What three changes have probably occurred in her eyes? What conditions or disease can develop in the aging person's vision? List three responses that will assist Mrs. Jones.

2. What is presbycusis? If your client has this condition, describe ways you can help the person compensate.

3. Mr. White is 85 years old. His appetite has been gradually decreasing and he has lost 10 pounds in the last month. What nursing measures could you take to help Mr. White enjoy his food more?

4. Explain why elderly people are more prone to develop hypothermia and hyperthermia. Identify a definite difference in the type of nursing assistant response given to these conditions.

5. Mrs. King tells you that the big toe on her left foot has a large blister. When you check the toe, Mrs. King tells you that she cannot feel your touch. What is the probable reason for her lack of sensitivity? What nursing responses should come to mind?

SUGGESTED ACTIVITIES

1. Participate in simulated sensory loss exercises provided by your instructor.
2. Participate in a classroom discussion of which sense you would miss the most and why. How would you like other people to respond to you?
3. Discuss behaviors of family members or friends who have sensory losses.
4. Visit agencies who offer treatment and/or training to those who are blind and deaf.
5. Invite a blind person to class to discuss his or her experiences and learn how you might improve your responses to the visually impaired.

CLINICAL APPLICATION

Select an elderly person with sensory loss for whom you give care, and using the checklist provided and using a problem-solving approach, provide nursing assistant responses to help compensate for the loss. Evaluate the results for any improvement after 2 weeks. Share the evaluation with your instructor, classmates, and staff.

WORKSHEET

Nursing Responses to Sensory Losses

Circle each number that applies to your client.

Place a check in the space if a response is given.

Nursing Responses:
<u>Compensation Measures</u>

I. Visual changes/visual acuity
1. Decreased visual acuity
2. Low tolerance for glare

_____ Eye exam; early treatment of eye diseases

_____ Provide quality lighting

_____ Avoid glare in environment

_____ Use hat to avoid sun

3. Low color distinction

_____ Provide gradual light changes

4. Poor adjustment to abrupt light changes

_____ Provide night lights

_____ Provide guardrails in halls and bathrooms

_____ Keep furniture away from doors

_____ Use large print, dials, and buttons on objects used frequently

_____ Provide color contrasts, not blended colors

_____ Leave furniture in the same place

_____ Provide assistance in dangerous areas

_____ Provide nonverbal communication: touch, hand-holding, patting, and so on

II. For persons with very poor vision and blind people

_____ Provide occupational therapy training

_____ Use textures to distinguish areas: fur handles on door, ticking clock to alert person to room; perfume smell to alert to room; satin pillowcase to alert to bed

_____ Use large calendars, clocks, and wall decorations at eye level

_____ Use "clock" method for feeding

_____ Have person close to TV set and to persons who are communicating

III. Auditory changes

1. Presbycusis—decrease in auditory acuity

_____ Speak clearly, close to the person

2. Men have more hearing loss

_____ Face person directly

3. Higher frequencies are the first to be lost

_____ Have light on your face so that the resident can see your lips

4. Sounds become distorted, heard incorrectly, and misinterpreted

_____ Use a lower voice; avoid high voice

5. Some people are irritated by music and noise

_____ Music played should have lower tones predominant

6. People with hearing aids should wear them; they need to be kept adjusted and worn properly

_____ Ask resident how they hear best

_____ Avoid background noise as much as possible; be alert to anxiety-producing noise

7. Hearing aids cannot help everyone

_____ Know how to care for and assist with hearing aids

8. The energy it takes to understand may be too much, and residents can easily withdraw.

_____ Use nonverbal communication, written messages, and so on

9. Paranoid tendencies and depression can easily occur with the hard of hearing since they do not know what is being said

_____ Provide opportunities that require less conversation: puzzles, reading, helping with food preparation, walks, outings

_____ Always inform residents what is going on, especially if he or she is present during a conversation

IV. Taste and smell
1. Decrease in taste and smell   _____ Provide colorful, tasteful food and verbal identification where vision is also a problem

2. Decreased nutrition due to inability to taste and enjoy   _____ Enjoyable mealtimes: pleasant surroundings, pleasant conversation

V. Temperature and touch: body, finger, and foot sensation

1. Decreased sensitivity to heat and cold   _____ Determine sensitivity status of client; provide proper garments

2. Circulatory disturbances, especially in long-term diabetics, which decreases sensitivity   _____ Always check on temperature of bath water, shower, and so on, especially if resident is self-care

_____ Additional protection: added warmth, foot care, and so on

Overall evaluation: (Include any additional specific responses and results)

_____

_____

_____

_____

4 ENVIRONMENTAL NEEDS OF THE ELDERLY

TERMINAL PERFORMANCE OBJECTIVE

Using a problem-solving approach, be able to assess a resident for environmental needs and provide the suggested compensatory measures to assist the client in achieving an optimal environment, one that assists the client to function in an improved and more independent way.

Enabling Objectives

1. Describe an optimal environment.
2. Give five examples of factors that create a poor environment.
3. List four environmental features of a nursing home which contribute to the independence of clients.
4. Describe how color can assist the visually impaired person.
5. Describe two features in the environment that meet the needs of wanderers.
6. Define *territoriality*.
7. Using a problem-solving approach, assist a client by providing compensatory measures in the environment.

REVIEW SECTION

It is suggested that nursing assistants taking this program of study should participate in a class discussion to review the variety of environments in nursing homes. Also review the positive and negative influences that the behavior of staff members can have on the environment.

UNDERSTANDING THE NURSING HOME ENVIRONMENT

According to writers who have studied the nursing home environment, most of the early nursing homes and those built in the early 1960s lacked provisions for the changes that occur in aging people. Many of these homes were built after the passing of the Medicare/Medicaid acts. These acts encouraged the building of nursing homes because funds were available to pay for some of the care. Little was known about how to adapt environmental design to meet older people's specialized needs. Not much attention was paid to the psychosocial needs of clients. Dignity, privacy, and the need to socialize were not considered. Today, more attention has been given to these needs and the effects that environment can have on a person's responses, especially the response to maintaining and promoting independent living.

THE RELATIONSHIPS AND EFFECTS OF THE ENVIRONMENT

The information provided in Units 2 and 3 helps to explain the expected negative effects that some environments will have on aging people. The aging person experiences a decreasing ability to adapt to change and stress that may be brought on by a change in environment. Loss of physical strength, induced by loss of muscle tissue and chronic disease, combined with psychosocial losses, such as loss of a spouse and home, tend to make an aging person vulnerable to environments that ignore the need to compensate for these losses. The vulnerable frail elderly person feels that the environment has control over his/her life. The geriatric nursing assistant is in a position to recognize the losses of each client and to provide compensatory measures that will give the client the opportunity to have some control.

When a person must give up his or her own home to enter a nursing home, many personal values are threatened. Privacy, a sense of security, and a place for keeping one's treasured items are suddenly taken away. It is therefore understandable that people in nursing homes will want to have some space to call their own. It becomes important to recognize the need for territoriality. Territoriality is often seen in animals, who serve as protectors of their owners and their territory by warding off other animals. Territoriality is also seen in humans, who try to assert their right to certain spaces and the items within them. The resident who is unhappy about someone else who has taken over his or her seat in the dining room is claiming territoriality.

The environment is also affected by the manner of the staff. If the staff members are warm and friendly and create an atmosphere wherein residents feel that they have dignity and a sense of equality and worth, you will find residents who have a sense of purpose and will want to be as independent as possible.

UNDERSTANDING THE ENVIRONMENTAL NEEDS OF RESIDENTS

Environments that are desired in nursing homes are those that provide devices to enable the person to be as mobile as possible. In other words, each person should be able to ambulate or to be as active as his or her condition allows. The geriatric health care team has an important role in evaluating the needs and potential of each client. Obviously, the physical therapist and occupational therapist contribute to this evaluation. The environment will necessitate that whatever devices are needed for each person will be available. These devices may include, but not be limited to, wheelchairs, walkers, crutches, canes, and other therapeutic appliances that promote independence and mobility (Figure 4.1).

Other environmental features that have importance to independence and control within the nursing home setting are the following: wider hallways and intersections to allow for the larger electronically controlled wheelchairs; wider doorways of rooms for wheelchair clearance; handrails in hallways and bathrooms; elevator buttons within reach of wheelchair-bound clients; lounges, bathrooms, and recreational areas clearly identified with large lettering and contrasting colors that help to identify separate areas; privacy rooms for clients and family members to visit without interruption; and lighting designed to compensate for the decrease in visual acuity. Other features are included in the checklist in this unit.

A supportive environment is equally important for the person with declining mental ability. Persons with memory impairment must have a safe environment that permits them to wander without fear of harming themselves or leaving the facility unnoticed. Color coding of doorways is one way of reminding residents where they are. The colors and what they represent must be reinforced by all staff. Pastel colors are not seen easily by aging clients; therefore, sharper, brighter colors are recommended. The use of large signs, calendars, and clocks also help to remind people of the activities scheduled, the time of day, and the day of the month. Providing only one entrance that is accessible to the wanderers, with a person placed to watch that entrance, provides an additional safety factor against a person leaving the building unnoticed. There should be a safe outdoor area for people of declining mental ability so that they can enjoy the outdoors.

Studies have indicated that if the environment matches a person's needs, the person exhibits a more positive self-concept. A person with a positive self-concept is more likely to strive for independence in living. It then becomes important for the geriatric nursing assistant to learn what can be provided in the environment that will match the client's needs and consequently support the person's positive self-concept and desire for independence.

The following checklist provides positive environmental features which have been found to assist elderly people in gaining more control while living in a nurs-

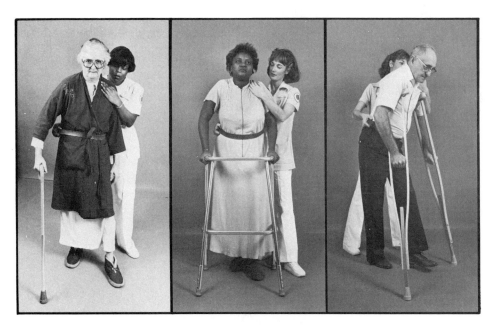

Figure 4.1. Mobility devices.

ing home. This checklist can be used to assess what might be lacking in the facility in which you work.

ENVIRONMENTAL CHECKLIST*

Directions: In doing an assessment of the facility in which you work, check off "yes" or "no" according to whether the desired feature is present.

Bathrooms

	Yes	No
1. Mirrors are placed or tilt so that people in wheelchairs can see themselves.	—	—
2. Lighting is bright but does not cause glare.	—	—
3. There is adequate space for manipulating a wheelchair through the doorways and into the stalls.	—	—
4. Doors close behind a person in a wheelchair.	—	—
5. A grab rail is available.	—	—
6. The sinks allow access for people in wheelchairs.	—	—
7. Towels, towel racks, and toilet paper are easy to reach.	—	—
8. Faucets are adapted for use by people with arthritic hands.	—	—
9. Call buttons are within easy reach.	—	—

Dining Room

1. Tables are high enough for wheelchairs to fit and to have easy access.	—	—
2. Tables have a nonglare surface and is a color that provides contrast with the plates and silverware.	—	—
3. The dining room is attractive and pleasant.	—	—
4. Lighting is bright enough without creating glare.	—	—
5. Windows have drapes or curtains so that glare can be eliminated.	—	—
6. There is a nice view and something to stimulate pleasant conversation.	—	—
7. Acoustics minimize noise from food carts and cafeteria/kitchen areas.	—	—
8. Chairs are sturdy, with arms, so that people can sit down and stand up independently.	—	—
9. Tables are small enough so that interaction is possible.	—	—

Accessibility/Mobility

1. Ramps provide wheelchair accessibility.	—	—
2. Elevator buttons are within the reach of wheelchair-bound people.	—	—

*Adapted with permission from the Ebenezer Center on Aging, Minneapolis, MN, *The Nursing Home Environment*, Kathy Carroll, Ed., 1978.

	Yes	*No*
3. There are handrails throughout the building at appropriate height.	—	—
4. Doors are light enough for older people to open.	—	—
5. Telephones are within reach of wheelchair-bound people.	—	—
6. Counters at the main desk or switchboard are low enough for wheelchair-bound people to get the attention of the person stationed there.	—	—

Visual Compensations

1. Light is adequate and falls on objects to be seen without glare.	—	—
2. There are adjustable window coverings.	—	—
3. Floors do not produce glare.	—	—
4. Carpets are plain or have very subtle patterns that do not give the illusion of obstacles to step over.	—	—
5. There is good ground contrast so that items in the environment can be seen.	—	—

Outdoor Areas

1. There is shelter from glare and sun.	—	—
2. Gardens and walkways are accessible, allow safe ambulation, and provide seating for tired people.	—	—
3. Walking surfaces enable people in wheelchairs to move their own wheelchairs.	—	—
4. There is some activity going on and a focal point that will promote conversation.	—	—
5. The texture and variety in plants/landscaping are appealing.	—	—

Bedrooms

1. Doorways are wide enough for wheelchairs.	—	—
2. The arrangement of furniture allows people to move about.	—	—
3. People have access to their own belongings.	—	—
4. Rooms are personalized.	—	—
5. People have their personal areas identified in each room.	—	—
6. There are curtains or some other device for assuring privacy.	—	—
7. Rooms are attractive.	—	—

Safety

1. All rugs lie flat.	—	—
2. There are no spills left on the floor; they are cleaned immediately.	—	—

	Yes	*No*
3. Cords from vacuum cleaners and other machines do not interfere with mobility and are clearly identified visually.	—	—
4. There are handrails throughout the facility.	—	—
5. Doors are not too heavy and do not close too fast.	—	—
6. Residents' rooms have furniture that is stable and will not roll away as a person uses it for balance.	—	—
7. There are no obstacles in the entranceway to rooms.	—	—
8. Hallways are free of clutter.	—	—
9. Furniture is not changed without the preference and knowledge of visually impaired people.	—	—

Promoting Family Involvement

1. Rooms are available for family parties and get-togethers.	—	—
2. Such things as a piano or a pool table are in the lounge area for family activity.	—	—
3. Schedules of activities are posted on bulletin boards with an invitation to families.	—	—
4. Outdoor areas include some playground equipment for children.	—	—
5. Small chairs, books, and magazines are provided for children who visit.	—	—
6. Picnic tables and chairs are provided for visiting with families.	—	—

Tactile Cues

1. Carpeting, wall surfaces, and furniture provide variety so that residents can determine environmental differences.	—	—
2. Bed linens, throw pillows, and curtains provide interesting textual qualities.	—	—
3. Tactile differences, such as fur pieces and carpet pieces, are used to assist visually impaired people to find their rooms and other items.	—	—
4. Differences in floor surfaces and wall surfaces are used to assist visually impaired people to identify areas or rooms.	—	—
5. Trees, bushes, and flowers are arranged so that people can be near them and touch them.	—	—

KEY POINTS

1. There are ways of compensating for sensory losses; these ways are often a matter of adjusting the environment.
2. Environmental adjustments need to become an integrated part of the care of each person.
3. A simple environmental adjustment, such as more light on the subject, can

often make the difference between the resident's capability for self-care and dependence on others.

4. This task was designed, in part, to help the geriatric nursing assistant be more keenly aware of the need to check the environment for obstacles and hazards that might retard the residents' independence.

SELF-CHECK

1. Mr. Willis is legally blind and walks with a cane. He always has difficulty finding the dining room. How can you help Mr. Willis without making him more dependent?

2. Newly admitted residents are often disoriented. What five environmental cues can you think of that would help ambulatory residents become oriented to the facility?

3. If Mrs. Brown is arguing with Mrs. Jones over who is to sit in the red chair, what need might they be exhibiting?

4. You are asked to be part of the team that will make suggestions for redesigning the recreational area. What suggestions would you make about the following: color scheme, lighting, and compensating features for the visually and hearing impaired. Consider measures learned from Unit 3.

5. Mr. Mahon has the declining mental abilities often seen in Alzheimer's disease. What environmental features should be provided so that he can walk about safely?

SUGGESTED ACTIVITIES

1. Visit several nursing homes to observe the different physical environments.
2. Talk to at least two residents for whom you do not give care about what they would like changed in the environment.

3. Visit a visually impaired person who lives at his or her own home to learn what adjustments had to be made in the environment.

4. Observe the differences in how staff members, including untrained nursing assistants, provide for residents' control of their environment. Report any differences to your class.

CLINICAL APPLICATION

Using the worksheet provided, select a resident for whom you give care, determine any environmental needs, and provide compensatory measures that will assist the resident to become more independent. Evaluate the resident regarding any improvement that may be made.

WORKSHEET

Environmental Checklist

	Yes	No
Bathrooms		
1. Mirrors are placed or tilt so that people in wheelchairs can see themselves.	—	—
2. Lighting is bright but does not cause glare.	—	—
3. There is adequate space for manipulating a wheelchair through the doorways and into the stalls.	—	—
4. Doors close behind a person in a wheelchair.	—	—
5. A grab rail is available.	—	—
6. The sinks allow access for people in wheelchairs.	—	—
7. Towels, towel racks, and toilet paper are easy to reach.	—	—
8. Faucets are adapted for use by people with arthritic hands.	—	—
9. Call buttons are within easy reach.	—	—
Dining Room		
1. Tables are high enough for wheelchairs to fit and to have easy access.	—	—
2. Tables have a nonglare surface and is a color that provides contrast with the plates and silverware.	—	—
3. The dining room is attractive and pleasant.	—	—
4. Lighting is bright enough without creating glare.	—	—
5. Windows have drapes or curtains so that glare can be eliminated.	—	—
6. There is a nice view and something to stimulate pleasant conversation.	—	—
7. Acoustics minimize noise from food carts and cafeteria/kitchen areas.	—	—
8. Chairs are sturdy, with arms, so that people can sit down and stand up independently.	—	—
9. Tables are small enough so that interaction is possible.	—	—
Accessibility/Mobility		
1. Ramps provide wheelchair accessibility.	—	—
2. Elevator buttons are within the reach of wheelchair-bound people.	—	—
3. There are handrails throughout the building at appropriate height.	—	—
4. Doors are light enough for older people to open.	—	—
5. Telephones are within reach of wheelchair-bound people.	—	—
6. Counters at the main desk or switchboard are low enough for wheelchair-bound people to get the attention of the person stationed there.	—	—
Visual Compensations		
1. Light is adequate and falls on objects to be seen without glare.	—	—

81

2. There are adjustable window coverings.   —   —

3. Floors do not produce glare.   —   —

4. Carpets are plain or have very subtle patterns that do not give the illusion of obstacles to step over.   —   —

5. There is good ground contrast so that items in the environment can be seen.   —   —

Outdoor Areas

1. There is shelter from glare and sun.   —   —

2. Gardens and walkways are accessible, allow safe ambulation, and provide seating for tired people.   —   —

3. Walking surfaces enable people in wheelchairs to move their own wheelchairs.   —   —

4. There is some activity going on and a focal point that will promote conversation.   —   —

5. The texture and variety in plants/landscaping are appealing.   —   —

Bedrooms

1. Doorways are wide enough for wheelchairs.   —   —

2. The arrangement of furniture allows people to move about.   —   —

3. People have access to their own belongings.   —   —

4. Rooms are personalized.   —   —

5. People have their personal areas identified in each room.   —   —

6. There are curtains or some other device for assuring privacy.   —   —

7. Rooms are attractive.   —   —

Safety

1. All rugs lie flat.   —   —

2. There are no spills left on the floor; they are cleaned immediately.   —   —

3. Cords from vacuum cleaners and other machines do not interfere with mobility and are clearly identified visually.   —   —

4. There are handrails throughout the facility.   —   —

5. Doors are not too heavy and do not close too fast.   —   —

6. Residents' rooms have furniture that is stable and will not roll away as a person uses it for balance.   —   —

7. There are no obstacles in the entranceway to rooms.   —   —

8. Hallways are free of clutter.   —   —

9. Furniture is not changed without the preference and knowledge of visually impaired people.   —   —

Promoting Family Involvement

1. Rooms are available for family parties and get-togethers.   —   —

2. Such things as a piano or a pool table are in the lounge area for family activity.   —   —

3. Schedules of activities are posted on bulletin boards with an invitation to families.   —   —

4. Outdoor areas include some playground equipment for children.   —   —

5. Small chairs, books, and magazines are provided for children who visit.   —   —

6. Picnic tables and chairs are provided for visiting with families.   —   —

	Yes	No
Tactile Cues		
1. Carpeting, wall surfaces, and furniture provide variety so that residents can determine environmental differences.	—	—
2. Bed linens, throw pillows, and curtains provide interesting textual qualities.	—	—
3. Tactile differences, such as fur pieces and carpet pieces, are used to assist visually impaired people to find their rooms and other items.	—	—
4. Differences in floor surfaces and wall surfaces are used to assist visually impaired people to identify areas or rooms.	—	—
5. Trees, bushes, and flowers are arranged so that people can be near them and touch them.	—	—

5 THE NEWLY ADMITTED ELDERLY RESIDENT

TERMINAL PERFORMANCE OBJECTIVE

Using information gathered from a newly admitted resident's reactions to nursing home admission, the reactions of his or her family members, and a problem-solving worksheet, be able to consider these reactions and provide geriatric nursing assistant responses to help the resident and family members to adjust.

Enabling Objectives

1. Explain why admission to a nursing home can be a critical time for an elderly person and his or her family members.
2. Discuss the effects that relocation may have on elderly people.
3. Describe two negative reactions that new residents might exhibit on being admitted to a nursing home.
4. List three prevailing psychological conditions that will help the nursing home resident accept admission to a nursing home.
5. Describe five nursing assistant approaches that are especially important when caring for a newly admitted elderly person.
6. List four nursing assistant approaches that are important when meeting family members of a newly admitted resident.
7. Provide geriatric nursing assistant responses that assist newly admitted clients and their family members to adjust to the nursing home.

REVIEW SECTION

The topics you should review with your instructor are the admission procedures for new residents and the emotional and psychological needs of the aging person.

A CRITICAL TIME

It has been well documented by sociologists and psychologists that relocation of an elderly person is for the most part a troubling experience. There is much controversy about how traumatic the experience is—whether it really has fatal effects on residents or not. It is clear that the adjustment to a nursing home can be unsettling and may develop into a crisis. Circumstances surrounding the move seem to make the difference between a fairly good adjustment and a poor one, according to W. Carole Chenitz (1983), a nurse who studied reactions of residents during the admission process. She found that some older people accept nursing home admission if they believe that it is necessary, it is the only reasonable choice, it is the result of their own decision, and if the stay will be for a short time. Older people who view the admission as undesirable, as a decision they did not make, and as a place where they will be permanently, usually will react against it. Chenitz also explained that the relocation of an elderly person from a comfortable secure environment, such as home, to the hospital for a critical illness, or to the nursing home for further care, can be an experience that will be far more serious than all other experiences.

The implication for the geriatric nursing assistant of the possible effects on a newly admitted elderly person is careful monitoring of the resident to see what behavior patterns are occurring. If the resident appears to be accepting, assistance is still needed. The resident will need help with coping and using whatever energy he or she has to make the adjustment. Looking at the psychosocial needs, not just the physical needs, is especially important at this time.

The resident who is "resisting" admission to a nursing home may exhibit challenging behaviors. If the resident begins to cry frequently, wants to stay in bed or in the bedroom, appears sad, or makes statements of helplessness, a crisis may be developing. It will require team conferences, utilizing everyone's skills, to help the resident accept admission when there are no other alternatives.

The elderly person who has been uprooted from a secure environment is usually suffering from more than relocation. Generally, the person has several chronic diseases, one or more of which may be in a more acute stage. Today, a person entering a nursing home from a hospital is a sicker person. With recent changes in the Medicare Act, hospitals are paid for Medicare patients by means of the prospective payment system, often referred to as DRG (for "diagnostic related groups"). The DRG system of payment reimburses hospitals for care based on the Medicare recipient's diagnosis, not on the total care provided. Hospitals, in turn, release patients based on that payment, whether or not they are ready to leave. Early release from hospitals puts people in nursing homes for their recuperating periods. These people are usually more acutely ill than was true of nursing home admissions in the past. If an elderly person is transferred from home to hospital, and then to a nursing home, several relocations occur, the effects of which can produce more stress on a person already stressed by illness.

People who experience sudden transfers have little time to adjust. The loss of a familiar environment is enough to cause confusion on the part of the older person who is experiencing the more subtle effects of the aging process discussed in Unit 2. It is not unusual for such a person to develop incontinence, to have jumbled speech, and to exhibit movements that may be interpreted as "senility" by those who do not know the person's previous habits. This type of confusion is often transitory and will clear when the person feels more secure.

NEED FOR FAMILY INVOLVEMENT

Involvement of family members can be crucial. Sometimes the resisting elderly person feels abandoned by the family. It is important for staff members to encourage visits from family members. These visits allow for the continuity of significant and familiar relationships and may help the elderly person feel more secure in the strange environment.

Family members have their own feelings to sort out at this time. Family members of resisting residents often feel guilty, frustrated, grief stricken, angry, and powerless. In these circumstances, assistance must be offered to family members as well, even to the extent of calling on mental health consultants. Not to resolve the crisis will mean that the resident will continue maladjusted and that family members will continue to harbor their own negative feelings.

Geriatric Nursing Assistant Responses

The geriatric nursing assistant spends more time with the new residents than does any other staff member. He or she can provide responses to the resident and to family members that will be most helpful. The following responses are recommended:

1. Greet the new person and family members with warmth and understanding. Introduce yourself. See figures 5.1(a) and 5.1(b).
2. Take time to listen to the concerns of resident and family. Report concerns that require other staff members' assistance.
3. If the resident is upset over the admission, get professional help immediately.
4. Allow the resident to have some control over decisions. Learn about personal choices from the resident and the family.
5. Encourage the resident to participate in self-care within the limits of safety.
6. Encourage the use of belongings and furnishings that personalize the room. Ask family members to bring in items.

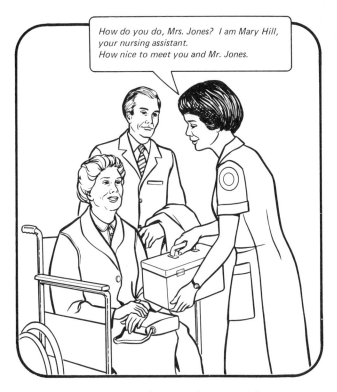

Figure 5.1(a). Greeting the new resident.

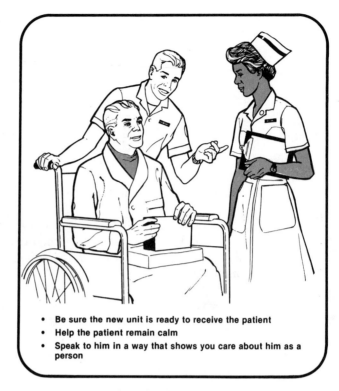

- Be sure the new unit is ready to receive the patient
- Help the patient remain calm
- Speak to him in a way that shows you care about him as a person

Figure 5.1(b).   Greeting the new resident.

7. Follow all admission procedures according to your facility. Be sure to orient the resident to the facility and to make introductions with other residents.

8. Identify needs and report these for incorporation into the plan of care. Seek suggestions from the family.

9. Determine if the new resident understands where he or she is. It may be necessary to tell the resident your name each time you come in contact with him or her. Provide reality orientation until the person is oriented. Report any signs of disorientation to the charge nurse. It will be necessary for all staff members to help with reality orientation.

10. Involve the resident in social activities as soon as possible or provide for continuation of the usual activities for the resident where feasible.

11. Remember that the nursing home is the resident's "home" now. Help to make it like a home environment: Protect the privacy and rights of each person; address each person with respect and dignity.

KEY POINTS

1. Admission to a nursing home or any change of location can be a crisis situation for a frail elderly person.

2. Complete assessment of all newly admitted residents is essential. Careful nursing care is needed to help prevent increased morbidity (illness) and mortality (death).

3. Protection of the resident's rights is essential to help maintain dignity, respect, and privacy.

4. Family members are important to the resident's well-being. They need assistance in adjusting to the nursing home admission of a loved one.

5. The nursing assistant is an integral part of the care team needed in the resident's and family's adjustment process.

SELF-CHECK

1. Mr. Bennett is 85 years old. He is recovering from a hip fracture. He is admitted from the hospital to your unit. Mr. Bennett has a catheter in place because "he was always incontinent of urine in the hospital." His daughter said that he was never incontinent before. What do you think might have caused Mr. Bennett's incontinence?

2. If Mrs. Smith is very quiet and withdrawn upon admission to the nursing home, what might be the cause of her reaction, and how would you go about trying to find out why she is acting this way?

3. Family members of Mr. Whitehead have not been to visit him since he was admitted 2 weeks ago. What reactions and feelings might the family members be having at this time? What feelings might Mr. Whitehead be having about not seeing them? What steps can you take to identify any problems?

4. Mrs. Hammond said to you: "I know I was put here to die." What strong feeling is she expressing? What nursing assistant actions can you take to try to help her?

5. The elderly person who adjusts best to a nursing home admission is one who has a part in the decision. What other factors contribute to a satisfactory adjustment?

SUGGESTED ACTIVITIES

1. Talk with at least two residents who have been in a nursing home for a year or more to learn how they felt on admission and how they feel now.
2. Visit an elderly person who is receiving care at home and ask the person how he or she feels about going to a nursing home if there was no one to help the person at home.
3. Have a conversation with an elderly member of your family about nursing homes. Note their reactions and feelings. Discuss these reactions in class.
4. Invite a family member who provides the care of an elderly person at home, or who has recently placed a loved one in a nursing home, to come to class to discuss feelings about the decisions that have to be made.

CLINICAL APPLICATION

Using the worksheet provided, interview an elderly person newly admitted to the nursing home and his or her family members, to determine reactions to the admission. Record on the worksheet the reactions and the nursing responses that are indicated. Include the titles of other team members who must be involved. Provide the responses for at least one week and evaluate the results.

WORKSHEET

**Interviewing a Newly Admitted Elderly Person and
Family Members**

Resident: _____   Diagnosis: _____
         (first name only)

General Description: (Describe the person by giving sex, age, physical limitations, general appearance, manner, emotions, etc.)

Person's reactions/feelings about admission: (Does she or he know how long they will stay? How did he or she decide to come to the nursing home? How can you best help him or her?)

Family members interviewed: (List the first names and relationships to elderly person.) What are the reactions/feelings about admission of their family member?

Geriatric nursing assistant responses indicated: (Include the other team members who must be involved.)

Evaluation: (What changes occurred after at least one week of nursing responses?)

6 COMMUNICATION IN THERAPEUTIC RELATIONSHIPS

TERMINAL PERFORMANCE OBJECTIVE

Be able to apply communication techniques, including the use of verbal, non-verbal, touch, humor, written, and telephone communications in the geriatric care facility.

Enabling Objectives

1. Identify six dimensions of a humanizing environment.
2. Identify the five parts of the communication process and their meanings.
3. Describe the basic foundations of a therapeutic relationship.
4. Describe five characteristics of effective communication.
5. List five barriers to effective communication.
6. Describe the precautions and benefits of humor and touch as forms of communication.
7. Identify five characteristics of effective written communication.
8. Identify five characteristics of effective telephone communication.
9. Apply effective techniques of communication (verbal, nonverbal, touch, humor, written, and telephone) in the geriatric care facility.

REVIEW SECTION

The topics to review with the instructor are the ways in which communication takes place in health care facilities and the responsibilities the nursing assistant has in communicating with clients, family members, team members, and supervising personnel.

Therapeutic relationships This unit will help you to improve your ability to communicate with residents, family members, and other members of the staff. Establishing therapeutic relationships means interacting with other people in such a way that the other person feels better and improves the way that he or she interacts in return. An example is the very quiet and withdrawn resident who eventually talks with you because of the way you have been able to help that person feel good about himself or herself again. Therapeutic relationships require a humanistic environment.

THE HUMANIZING ENVIRONMENT

It has been noted, especially by professionals who work on rehabilitation teams, that one of the most important elements of a therapeutic and humanizing environment is an atmosphere of expectancy of improvement. The emotional tone of the staff must reflect respect to the client so that the client is made to feel capable of recovering. This tone conveys a feeling that the person is valued and helps to establish a sense of confidence.

There are other dimensions of respect that need to be conveyed to residents in nursing homes if they are to feel they are being treated as human beings. These dimensions include:

1. A sense that he or she is different in a special way and not like any other person
2. A sense that he or she is a person with a lifetime of experiences, a holistic person who has feelings, actions, and attitudes and should not be pulled apart by different specializing professionals
3. Some freedom to choose, especially in regard to one's own care
4. A feeling of being treated as an equal and not as subservient to the staff
5. A sense of empathy coming from the staff and an opportunity to be empathetic in return
6. A sense that staff view him or her as a human being with feelings and not as a diagnosis or nonperson
7. Confidence that he or she is not a source of sick humor for the staff to laugh about and cajole for their own pleasure

Episodes of severe dehumanization and depersonalization have occurred in nursing homes and still occur. It is essential that the geriatric nursing assistant contribute to the humanizing environment in daily interactions with staff, residents, and family members. See figures 6.1(a) and 6.1(b).

IMPLEMENTING THE PHILOSOPHY OF CARE

In Unit 1 you learned that a sound philosophy of care is one that is humanistic and holistic. The dimensions above provide a more specific way of looking at that philosophy as it is applied in daily interactions with residents. Implementing the philosophy simply means that you apply the dimensions to each person and staff member as you give care to residents and as you work with the staff. You will find that when each staff member believes and applies this philosophy, residents will know that you and other staff members care and want the very best for them. You will also find residents who want to improve.

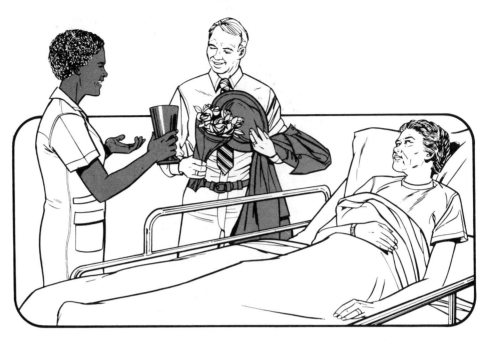

Figure 6.1(a).   Friendly communication with family members.

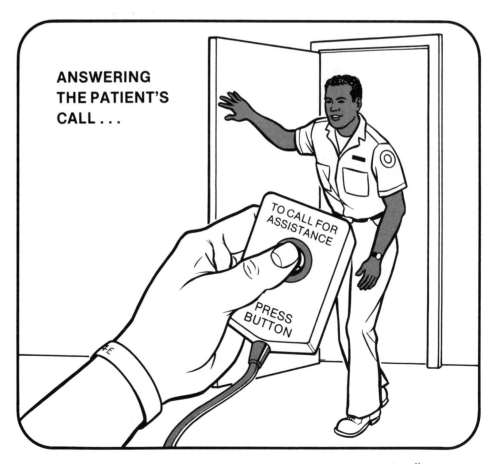

Figure 6.1(b).   Respond promptly to the resident's or patient's call.

BASIC FOUNDATIONS OF RELATIONSHIPS

The ability of the geriatric nursing assistant to be able to communicate and to build satisfactory relationships cannot be overemphasized. Communication is the basis for all human understanding, interactions, and relationships. Communication can be spoken or verbal, or nonverbal (gestures, signals, facial and body expressions), or written, as in the plan of care. Communication is defined as a means of sending and receiving messages. The communication process, although described many ways by different people, involves five parts.

1. *Sender:* person initiating the message
2. *Transmitting medium:* method used to convey the message
3. *Message:* words spoken, written, gestures, or other symbols; the thoughts and ideas conveyed by the sender
4. *Receiver:* person to whom the message is intended
5. *Feedback:* evidence that the receiver understands the message

Unfortunately, feedback is not requested enough by persons sending messages and becomes a major reason why the communication process breaks down. For example, you are giving directions to someone about how to find the nursing home:

Sender: "Go down Main Street until you reach the greenhouse and turn right. There is only one greenhouse, so you can't miss the turn."
Receiver: understands he is looking for a green house (colored green); never sees one, so misses the turn.
Undelivered message: the greenhouse: a building made of glass that houses flowers.
Feedback: not clarified, not requested.

Feedback is very important when working with the elderly because of the losses in hearing, vision, touch, and other senses. Caregivers who do not take the time to assess the older person's ability to understand the message will have a breakdown in communication.

The geriatric nursing assistant who can help the elderly feel good about themselves has a priceless gift. The geriatric nursing assistant communicates with clients on a daily basis and therefore develops interpersonal relationships, relationships that involve a sharing of ideas and feelings. Effective relationships evolve from two basic foundations: trust and rapport. Trust requires confidence in another person, a feeling that another person will act in your best interest, and these actions are favorable and predictable. Rapport develops from trust. Rapport means to be in agreement or in harmony with another person. You know that you have an effective interpersonal relationship when you trust the other person and have established rapport; a feeling of comfort exists when sharing your thoughts and concerns without fear of being criticized, embarrassed, or the subject of gossip. Confidentiality is an essential part of an effective relationship (Figure 6.2).

Confidentiality is also a right of each client and must be respected at all times. Confidentiality means that all matters pertaining to information about clients is secret and is not discussed with anyone who is not privileged to know it. Discussion of clients is necessary with other team members and care givers involved in the plan of care. However, to discuss information about clients with your own family or friends is violating the client's right to confidentiality. The geriatric

ETHICS OF CONFIDENTIALITY

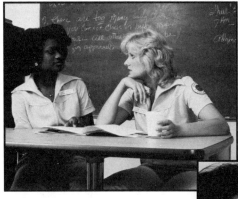

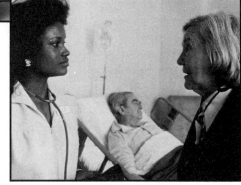

DO NOT DISCUSS PATIENT INFORMATION WITH

- ONE PATIENT ABOUT ANOTHER PATIENT
- RELATIVES AND FRIENDS OF THE PATIENT
- VISITORS TO THE HOSPITAL
- REPRESENTATIVES OF NEWS MEDIA
- FELLOW WORKERS, EXCEPT WHEN IN CONFERENCE
- YOUR OWN RELATIVES AND FRIENDS

Figure 6.2. Ethics of confidentiality.

nursing assistant must guard that right. A breach of confidentiality can be a reason for a lawsuit as well as a reason for poor relationships.

VERBAL AND NONVERBAL TECHNIQUES OF COMMUNICATION

Effective spoken communication is clearly understood between the sender and the receiver. It requires active listening on the part of the receiver. Active listening means that the listener is receiving the entire message—the words and the feelings that are being expressed. An example of active listening: After asking Mrs. Smith how she feels today, she replies in a very sad voice, "I'm fine." She obviously isn't fine because you detected sadness in her voice. Noting the sadness means that you were actively listening to the tone of her voice, which conveyed a different message than the words spoken. Active listening also includes observation of the nonverbal behavior during the communication.

Techniques of verbal communication, besides active listening, which the geriatric nursing assistant should apply are the following:

1. Speech is clear.
2. Vocabulary is understood by clients.
3. A nonverbal response, such as a nod of head, is provided to indicate understanding.
4. The message is clarified by giving back main points said by client.
5. The message is rephrased back to the client as another way to make sure that you understand.
6. The client is allowed to express anger and hostile behavior. (Do not try to cut off behavior that you do not like.)
7. A calm touch on the client's hand or shoulder is used when appropriate. (*Note:* Touch the person's hand first; some people do not like to be touched.)
8. Eye contact is maintained with the client.
9. The speaker is given time to finish—do not hurry or appear distracted.
10. The client is spoken to with respect and as an equal.

A checklist will help guide you in your verbal and nonverbal communications.

CHECKLIST FOR COMMUNICATION: VERBAL AND NONVERBAL

	Yes	No
1. Listens carefully for feelings as well as words.	—	—
2. Uses eye contact during the conversation.	—	—
3. Shows sensitivity to feelings.	—	—
4. Tone of voice is appropriate.	—	—
5. Verbal and nonverbal responses are appropriate in choice of words and gestures.	—	—
6. Uses silence when appropriate.	—	—
7. Gives time for respondent to answer.	—	—
8. Clarifies what the message is.	—	—
9. Repeats important words or ideas of respondent.	—	—
10. Uses open-ended sentences, avoiding yes-and-no answers.	—	—
11. Uses touch and other nonverbal techniques when appropriate.	—	—
12. Avoids judgments or value statements.	—	—
13. Summarizes, using respondent's words to help clarify the message.	—	—

BARRIERS TO COMMUNICATION

Barriers to communication are those actions that prevent effective communication. Some of the barriers that the geriatric nursing assistant should avoid are:

1. Labeling or stereotyping people because of preset ideas and prejudices
2. Allowing yourself to become angry about the client's words or behavior
3. Speaking to the older person in a demeaning or childish manner

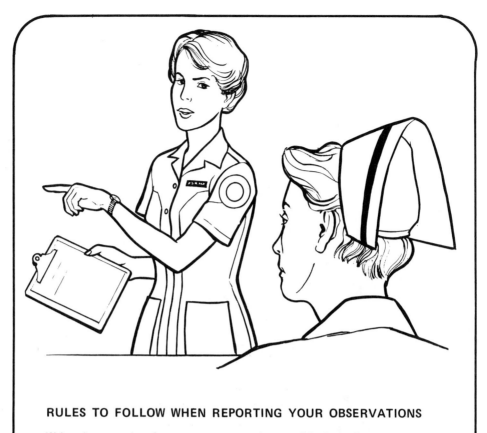

RULES TO FOLLOW WHEN REPORTING YOUR OBSERVATIONS

Write down patient's name, room number, and bed number
Write or report your observations to the head nurse or team leader as
  soon as possible
Report the time you made the observation
Report the location of the abnormal or unusual sign
Report exactly, but report only what you observe, that is,
  report objectively

Figure 6.3(a). Rules for reporting observations.

4. Interrupting the speaker—interjecting your own ideas
5. Making value statements about the client's beliefs, telling him or her what they believe is wrong
6. Talking too fast or too low so that the client cannot hear you
7. Making jokes out of clients' expressions of feeling unhappy or upset
8. Using medical terms that the client cannot understand
9. Ignoring the need for an interpreter when a client cannot understand the spoken language of the country
10. Giving false reassurances—telling clients they will be fine when they are actually terminally ill

People who have studied the process of communication believe that non-verbal expressions are far more important than the spoken word. When you take time to think about how much we use gestures and facial expressions to say what we mean and feel, it is easy to understand the meaning and importance of non-verbal behavior. An effective caregiver must learn to use nonverbal behavior appropriately. This means learning acceptance of: disfigurement, hostile behaviors, odors from foul-smelling wounds or diseased parts of the body, and similar conditions which may cause facial and body expressions that offend clients. On the other hand, it is through facial expression that we can show empathy, concern, interest, and happiness when caring for clients. Figures 6.3(a) and 6.3(b) show how to report your nonverbal observations.

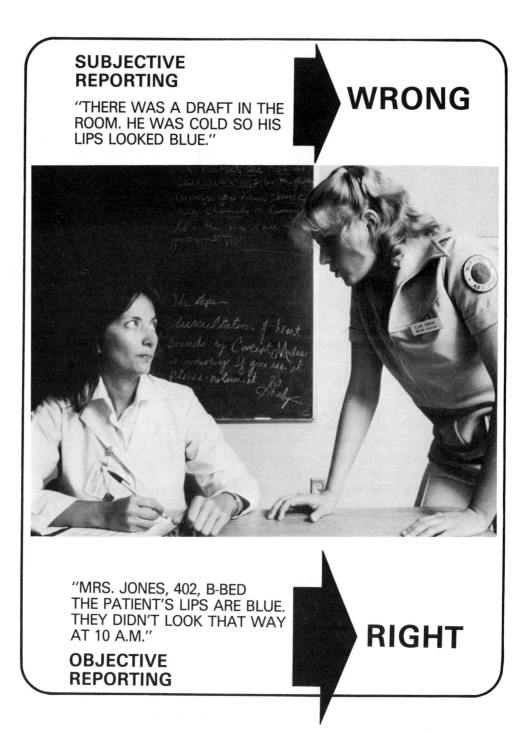

Figure 6.3(b).   Correct reporting of nonverbal behavior.

THE BENEFITS OF TOUCH AND HUMOR

Touch

The use of touching has been shown to be very important in nursing. See figures 6.4(a), 6.4(b), and 6.4(c). Some nurses have used touch in the form of therapy for calming highly anxious patients on psychiatric and cardiovascular units. Other nurse researchers have found that a systematic program of using touch in the daily care of patients actually improves individuals' states of health physiologically and psychologically.

It is generally agreed that the aging person who is progressively losing the ability to see and hear needs an increase in tactile stimulation, or more touching. Touching for these people is a form of communication that can have harmful effects as well as positive ones. It is therefore very important for the caregiver to use a calm, soothing manner when touching, which can be interpreted as a sign of caring, rather than a rough manner, interpreted as uncaring and abusive.

Caution must be taken to assess the elderly person's acceptance of touch. People of different cultures have different tolerance levels of touching. It is recommended that a hand be extended to an individual first before offering more intimate forms of touching, such as hugging. Hugging is a form of touch that is much more enthusiastic and apparently more therapeutic than hand-holding or a pat on the back. Some researchers have called hugging a miracle medicine, saying that a full embrace is sometimes helpful in: relieving pain, living longer, curing depression and stress, strengthening family relationships, and in helping a person to sleep. Hugging has also been named as a factor in raising the body's

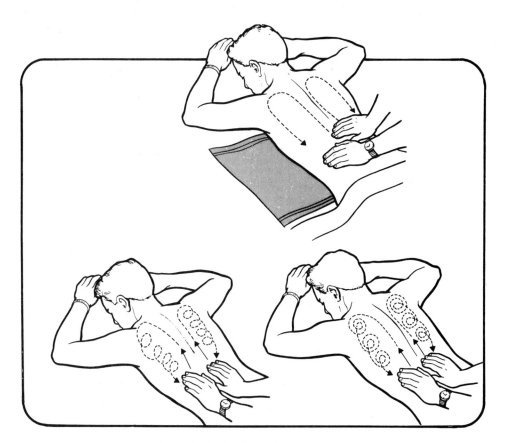

Figure 6.4(a). The backrub is a form of therapeutic touch.

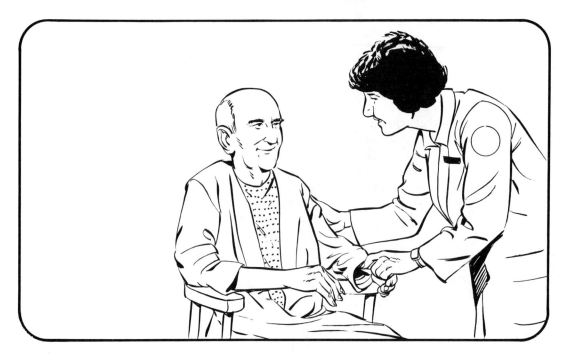

Figure 6.4(b).   Non-threatening ways to touch.

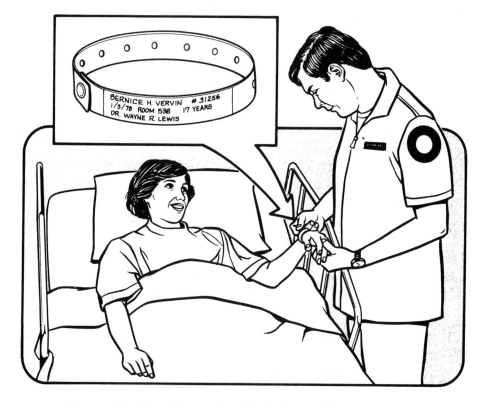

Figure 6.4(c).   Touch the resident's hand when in doubt about how to touch.

hemoglobin level. Hemoglobin is the iron-containing protein pigment of the blood that carries oxygen to all organs of the body. A normal hemoglobin level is essential to a feeling of well-being and aids in the recovery from illness. A decreased hemoglobin level is not uncommon among elderly people. It should make us wonder if more hugging and touching would help more residents in nursing homes feel and act as though they were in the prime of life.

Irene Burnside, a nurse researcher who has devoted many years to working with the elderly, developed guidelines about incorporating touch into the client's plan of care. The essence of her guidelines for incorporating touch into daily care is summarized here.

Provide increased touching when:

1. The person is becoming more isolated because of losses: in sensorium, of loved ones, of self-esteem, of body image due to disfigurement, and because of fear of approaching death.
2. The person is becoming more withdrawn and is not talking.
3. The person is more anxious and needs to be calmed.

Be cautious with touch when:

4. The person wants more privacy.
5. The person has a great need for territoriality.

Humor

Humor is often related to something that is amusing or that which is funny and entertaining. Humor may be described as the circumstance that caused the laughter or the response to what was humorous. Other responses to humor can be smiling or a feeling within us that says we have been amused. Sometimes a feeling of relaxation is a response to humor. Regardless of how we define it, or how we respond to it, humor has been awarded many benefits. The reaction of laughter has been called "internal jogging" because of the physiological responses that are actually benefits to the body similar to the benefits of jogging. The body systems and the benefits are:

> *Respiratory system:* increased respiratory rate and increased oxygen exchanges
> *Musculatory system:* increased muscular activity, which also increases the heart rate and stimulates the heart muscle
> *Nervous system:* increased production of catecholamines, which stimulate the production of endorphins, the body's natural pain-reducing enzyme

The relief of pain from laughter gained national recognition with Norman Cousins' book in 1979 on *The Anatomy of An Illness*. Cousins documented the relief of severe pain for at least 2 hours following 10-minute sessions of humorous films accompanied by massive doses of vitamin C.

Other benefits of humor and laughter as a response include: relief of stress through relaxation, outlets for anger, escape from an unbearable situation, and a means of coping in times of difficulty.

Registered nurses have formed an organization called Nurses For Laughter (NFL). These nurses believe in its benefits. Guidelines have been suggested for the use of humor when using it to help clients. The guidelines are helpful to geriatric nursing assistants when working with the elderly. They are in the form of a checklist.

CHECKLIST FOR USE OF HUMOR

	Yes	*No*
1. The time for humor is appropriate.	—	—
2. There is no chance of misunderstanding.	—	—
3. The client is in a playful mood and receptive.	—	—
4. The humor is not offensive.	—	—

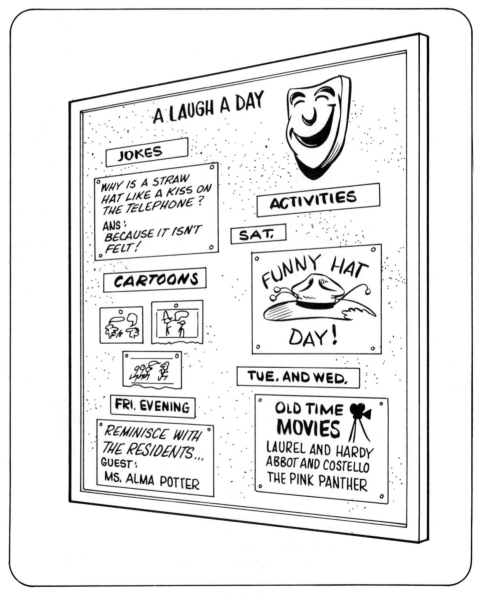

Figure 6.5. Humor is therapeutic.

	Yes	No
5. The content is understood to be humorous.	—	—
6. There are verbal or nonverbal cues that what is said is a joke. ("I have a story to tell you," or a wink/smile to indicate a joking mood that is clearly understood.)	—	—
7. The receiver is not in pain and is able to take part in the humor.	—	—

Humor has been studied in nursing homes by the Andrus Gerontology Center in California. Some of the benefits they found for the residents, after a series of planned humorous events, included: renewed interest in social activities, more smiles and laughter, increase in positive-outgoing attitudes, and initiation from some of the residents in planning their own activities.

The role of providing events for residents in nursing homes usually belongs to the activity or recreational therapist. As a team member, the geriatric nursing assistant can be a "humor advocate." Humor provides a relaxed, happy atmosphere if used appropriately and according to the guidelines. Consider how much more fun it would be going to work where your residents are involved and happy and ready to have some laughter. You can build a reservoir of jokes, cartoons, funny one-liners, and other ideas to provide laughter in your caregiving (Figure 6.5).

WRITTEN COMMUNICATIONS

The amount of written communication the geriatric nursing assistant does in a nursing home varies from one nursing home to another. However, knowing how to do good reporting and charting should be valued by every nursing assistant. One way to organize your thoughts for reporting the care you have given is to follow a basic outline which includes: the identified need, signs and symptoms, nursing assistant actions taken, and the results of the actions.

An example of the outline as it applies to a resident in a nursing home is given below.

Need	Signs/Symptoms	Actions	Results
Difficulty walking	Right knee stiff and swollen due to arthritis	Assisted with walker	Walked 20 feet, 5 feet more than yesterday

The geriatric nursing assistant can organize his or her thoughts in this way and be prepared to report them orally or in writing. To be organized takes practice but the more you practice, the easier it is and then it becomes automatic.

Charting on the resident's chart means writing notes on a legal document. The chart can be called into a courtroom if there is a lawsuit about the care given. It is therefore important that the geriatric nursing assistant writes any notes on a separate piece of paper and has them checked by the nurse in charge before writing on the chart. The characteristics of effective written communication in the following checklist should be applied to all charting.

CHECKLIST FOR CHARTING

	Yes	No
1. The writing form used (print or manuscript) and color of ink are according to facility policy.	—	—
2. Words are clear, legible, and spelled correctly.	—	—
3. Care given reflects needs, signs/symptoms, actions, and results.	—	—
4. Errors are crossed through with one line, marked "Error" and initialed. (Do not erase or white out with fluid.)	—	—
5. All written entries have time, date, and are signed.	—	—
6. All entries are made after care is given and not before.	—	—
7. The person giving the care makes the entry and signs it.	—	—
8. Abbreviations used are according to facility policy.	—	—

TELEPHONE COMMUNICATIONS

The telephone is an important line of communication in any health care facility. You are representing the caregivers in your nursing home when you talk to the public. This kind of communication comes under the category of "public relations." How you respond is very important to the image created in the minds of people who call.

It is essential that you be tactful and diplomatic but also friendly. The tone of voice should be pleasant and reflect a "smile on your face." A high screeching voice should be avoided. A moderate tone using clear and distinct words is best.

The telephone should be answered promptly, at least by the second ring. Always identify the facility and yourself: "Good morning, Capital Nursing Home, Miss Jones speaking. May I help you?" is a pleasant way to answer the phone. You immediately let the caller know if they have the right place/person. When speaking on the phone, it is best to keep the mouthpiece about 1 inch from your lips.

In taking messages, it is necessary to ask who is calling and request spelling of the person's name when in doubt. Paper and pencil should always be by the telephone to take down the following information: name of caller, full telephone number with the area code if out of state, date and time of call, summary of the message, and any action taken. Always sign or initial the message so that the person called can request additional information if the message is unclear.

Sometimes discretion is needed on the part of the person taking the call. If the person being called is in a conference or with a resident, you can say, "Miss Jones is busy now, may I take a message and have her return your call?" Always say "thank you for calling" as you conclude the call. If a person is put on hold, be sure to get back to the person and apologize for having him or her wait. It is necessary to show consideration to all callers no matter how unpleasant the caller might be. Be sure to check on your facility policies regarding unpleasant callers. Usually, the supervisor or administrator will respond to people who are unhappy about a situation.

It is your responsibility to know how to respond to personal calls. Generally, staff members are not to make or accept personal calls while on duty. Check with your supervisor and know the policies of the facility. The following checklist is one that you can use to practice taking messages while on duty.

CHECKLIST FOR TELEPHONE COMMUNICATION

	Yes	No
1. Uses friendly voice with a "smile."	—	—
2. Identifies self and institution with "May I help you?"	—	—
3. Uses moderate tone; avoids high, screeching voice.	—	—
4. Answers telephone promptly (by second ring).	—	—
5. Holds receiver about 1 inch from lips.	—	—
6. Takes complete message: name, telephone number, message summary, date, time, action taken, initials form.	—	—
7. Uses discretion if person called is busy.	—	—
8. Promptly returns to caller if caller placed on "Hold."	—	—
9. Follows policy if caller is irate or angry.	—	—
10. Completes call by saying "Thank you for calling."	—	—

KEY POINTS

1. Nonverbal communication is considered more important than spoken communication because we use it almost 100 percent of the time.
2. Geriatric nursing assistants are with the clients more than other staff members; therefore, effective communication skills are of primary importance; feedback must be requested.
3. Humor and touch are two more tools that can become effective communication techniques when used appropriately. They also benefit the client physiologically and psychologically.
4. The resident's chart is a legal document; it must be accurate and complete.
5. The geriatric nursing assistant represents the facility when answering the telephone. Telephone communication skills are a valuable part of effective communications.

SELF-CHECK

1. Identify six dimensions of a humanizing environment.
2. What is essential in the communication process to assure that the message is understood?
3. Describe a trusting relationship.
4. What characteristics contribute to effective communications? What are the barriers?
5. You want to try some humor with Mr. Brown, who rarely smiles. How would you proceed?
6. Mrs. Holder is quiet today and seems very sad. How would you proceed to use touch as a form of communication?
7. You took care of "Annie" (her favorite name) today. Annie has had a broken hip and is beginning to walk. Using the suggestions and the checklist for charting, write nursing notes about how Annie walked today. (You will need to make up what activity Annie had.)
8. A son of John Jones called to say how upset he was that his father's teeth

looked so dirty when he visited last evening. You answered the telephone. How would you answer the phone, and how would you respond to the son?

SUGGESTED ACTIVITIES

1. Practice communication techniques with classmates. Use the checklist as your guide.

2. Observe communication at home between your relatives. Identify good and poor techniques. What seemed to be the main problem when poor techniques were used?

3. Analyze why you trust someone and compare your reasons with the residents' relationships you have. Why do some residents want to do what you ask, and why do others not want to?

4. Discuss in class how you feel about humor and touch.

5. Invite a person from the telephone company to talk about telephone communications and what he or she has to recommend about telephone techniques.

CLINICAL APPLICATION

1. Residents who need assistance with their care are described on the worksheet provided. Read about each one and then practice charting nursing notes, remembering to include the need, signs/symptoms, actions taken, and results. When writing notes you do not write the words need, signs/symptoms, and so on. You keep the outline in your mind as you write. See the example below. Use the checklist provided in this unit to guide you when you write your notes. Have your instructor check your notes.

    Example:

    2/20/88   Resident has difficulty walking d/t arthritis of the rt. knee.
    10:00A.   Knee is swollen (14 inches in circumference) and very stiff. Assisted with walker. Resident walked 20 feet today, 5 feet farther than yesterday. Tolerance for activity is improving.

    D. Witmer, GNA

    Abbreviations allowed by facility: d/t = due to; rt. = right

2. Complete the worksheet provided to use when applying the techniques of verbal, nonverbal, touch, and humor. Select a resident, then apply the guidelines for touch and humor and the checklist for verbal and nonverbal communications. Report on the results to your instructor and classmates. Share with the staff within your work setting.

3. Complete the worksheet "Telephone Communications." Use the checklist in this unit as a guide.

WORKSHEET

Written Communications

1. Mrs. Jones is on range of motion to the left arm. She had a broken humerus (bone in the upper arm) 3 months ago.

2. Mr. Green has had severe constipation. A slice of bran bread has been incorporated in his meals three times a day to alleviate this condition.

3. Mr. Black has had pneumonia and is slowly ambulating again. His respirations were up to 40 per minute when he first started to walk after his illness.

WORKSHEET

Verbal and Nonverbal Communications

Resident: _____ Communication techniques: _____
(first name only)
                                   Conversation:

_____

Verbal: words spoken, humor used. (Write what you said and what the resident said.)

Nonverbal: gestures, facial expression, body movements, touch used. (Write any nonverbal expressions used by you and the resident.)

Interpretation: Write what you think took place during the conversation. (Did the resident feel better after the communication?) How could you do better next time?

WORKSHEET

Telephone Communications

Your Name: _____ Facility Name: _____

Conversation:

_____

What you said: What person calling said:

Interpretation: Write what you think took place during the conversation. Were there any problems? Did you follow the checklist? Did someone else have to be called to the phone?

7 *INFECTION CONTROL AND ACCIDENT PREVENTION*

Infection Control

TERMINAL PERFORMANCE OBJECTIVE

Given information and review of infection control measures, characteristics of aging residents who are prone to infections, and skill checklists on handwashing, gloving, and donning and removing isolation gowns and masks, be able to apply infection control measures.

Enabling Objectives

1. Identify the responsibilities geriatric nursing assistants have in daily infection control.
2. Define medical asepsis.
3. Describe three requirements for organisms to grow.
4. Describe five times when hand washing should be done.
5. Define nosocomial infection.
6. Explain why the geriatric nursing assistant must be concerned with the transmission of AIDS in a health care setting.
7. Explain why elderly people are susceptible to infection.
8. List and describe the six universal precautions to be taken by all health care workers to prevent transmission of HIV (human immunodeficiency virus).
9. Practice skills in handwashing and in application and removal of gloves, gowns, and masks.

REVIEW SECTION

The topics the geriatric nursing assistant should review with the instructor are infection control measures, including principles of isolation.

IMPORTANT WORDS TO UNDERSTAND

Experienced nursing assistants should be able to correctly use key words in infection control and have the basic knowledge, proper attitude, and skills for assisting with infection control. *Asepsis* means free of pathogenic or disease-producing organisms (Figure 7.1). *Medical asepsis* is a term that means prevention of

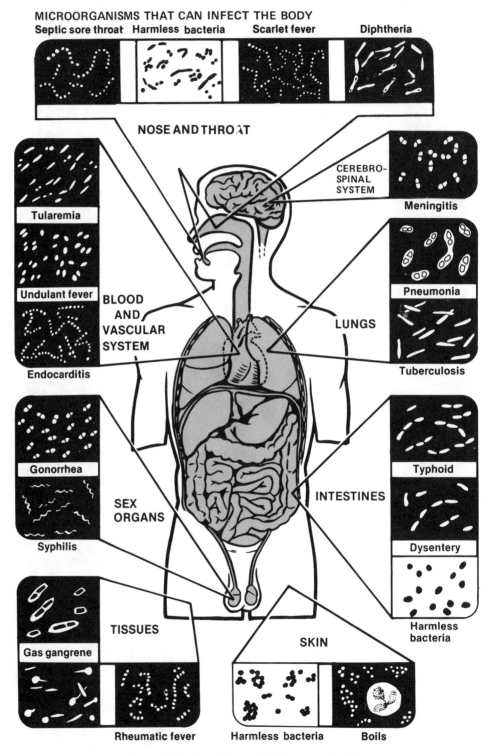

Figure 7.1. Conditions affecting growth of bacteria.

the spread of disease by getting rid of organisms through everyday cleaning practices. Handwashing, bathing, and general cleaning are practices of medical asepsis. *Surgical asepsis*, on the other hand, are those practices that eliminate all organisms, such as sterilizing with use of the autoclave. Organisms grow in environments that have moisture, warmth, and nourishment (Figure 7.2). The objective of all aseptic techniques is to prevent an environment conducive to the growth of organisms. By following infection control measures in daily activity, the geriatric nursing assistant is a valuable contributor to the prevention of infection in elderly clients.

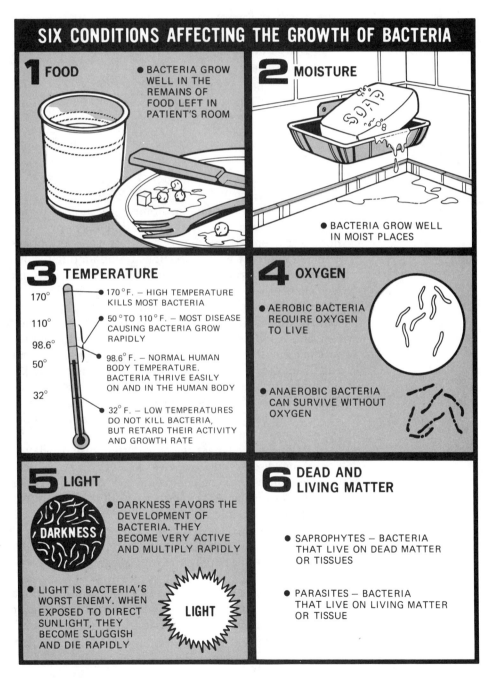

Figure 7.2.

SPECIAL CONSIDERATIONS WITH THE ELDERLY

The elderly person is prone to more infections as aging changes occur. In general, the aging person has less resistance to infection because of a deficient immune system. Normally functioning immune systems ward off infection or bring it under control fairly quickly. Changes occur at variable rates for the elderly, so the amount of resistance will be different for each person. Antibodies, which help to fight certain organisms, also decrease with age.

Some diseases and conditions that predispose the elderly to infections, according to Smith, are:*

Diabetes mellitus
Congestive heart failure
Dehydration
Malnutrition
Immobility
Hospitalization
Diminished pain sensitivity symptoms
Decreased mental ability (unable to describe illness)
Tumors
Drugs

The elderly in nursing homes are subject to nosocomial infections. A nosocomial infection is an infection that develops while a person is in a nursing home (or hospital). Studies of infection rates in nursing homes indicate a rate of 2 to 15 percent. Most infections found among residents have been due to infected decubiti, conjunctivitis, cystitis/pyelonephritis, pneumonia, diarrhea, and influenza.

Some residents who have infections may not receive treatment. The problem with residents receiving no treatment may be due to the way that elderly residents respond to the presence of infections in their bodies. Because an elderly resident may have several underlying diseases, the acute phase of an infection can be masked and missed. Fever, which is normally present in younger people with infections and is an early indication of infection, may not be present in the elderly person. The elderly person is also frequently receiving medications such as aspirin or steroids for other diseases. These medications keep the temperature from rising.

Additional changes in the elderly cause a delayed diagnosis. Besides the underlying diseases, the elderly experience decreased sensitivity to pain and may develop confusion. The confusion may cause the person to be unable to truly describe the effects of the infection. Both the sensation of pain and a clear mental state are factors in the elderly that are needed to alert the care giver of any problems that the elderly person may have.

Other age-related changes in elderly residents predispose them to infections. These changes are mainly the following:

1. Difficulty is encountered with fluid and nutritional maintenance. Loss of adequate fluids leads to diminished urinary flow and mucus production in the respiratory tract; consequently, these organs can become infected.
2. The skin, which is the first line of defense against invasion by organisms,

*From P. W. Smith, ed., *Infection Control in Long Term Care Facilities*, Wiley, New York © 1984. Reprinted by permission of John Wiley & Sons, Inc.

loses fat and becomes thin; prevention of pressure areas and skin tearing becomes a high priority.

3. Gastric acid decreases, thereby diminishing the protective action of the acid against gastrointestinal infections.

4. Urinary tract is susceptible to infection, especially with decreased urinary flow and the presence of catheters.

5. The respiratory tract may have a decreased cough reflex and less mucus, due to dehydration or medication. Prevention of aspiration into the lung is essential to avoid pneumonia.

General measures of nursing care must focus on the adequate hydration, ambulation, and documentation of skin conditions and catheter care of residents. Daily cleanliness of the skin and at least several baths a week have been recommended. Particular attention to the perineal area of residents must be given to avoid the accumulation of more persistent bacteria and subsequent excoriation. Excoriated skin (redness and abrasion of skin) is a predisposing condition for skin infection. Figure 7.3 shows how infections can be transmitted in a health

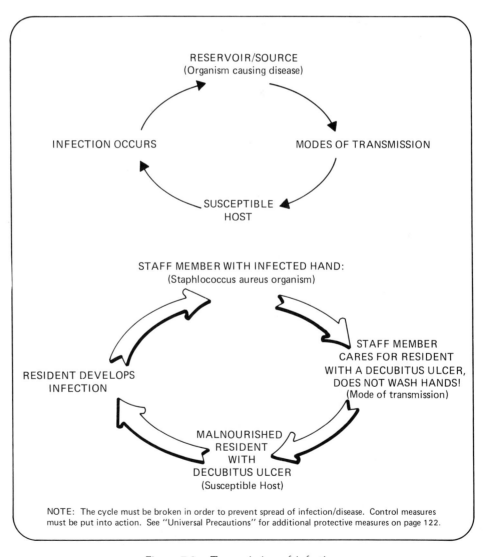

Figure 7.3. Transmission of infection.

care setting. The cycle shown must be broken to prevent the spread of infection/disease. Control measures must be put into action. See "Universal Precautions to Prevent HIV Transmission" for additional protective measures. The geriatric nursing assistant can respond by following the methods suggested below.

Nursing responses to control infection at the source

1. Maintain health; have illnesses and infections treated. Report any breaks in your skin, especially hands.
2. Do not attend residents when you are ill or infected. Notify the supervisor of any infections.
3. Carry out handwashing, following the technique recommended.
4. Follow policies for disinfection and sterilization.
5. Do your part in housekeeping.
6. Fold and carry clean and dirty linen properly.
7. Dispose of soiled disposable articles properly.

Nursing responses to control infection at the transmission level

1. Carry out handwashing before and after caring for residents (see box on p. 121–122).
2. Follow policies on catheter care.
3. Follow aseptic technique in caring for residents and in disposing of articles. Follow universal precautions.
4. If several residents have the same symptoms, determine the means of transmission and intervene to prevent transmission where possible. Wash your hands!
5. Become informed and inform residents of how to prevent infections and illnesses.
6. Wipe up any spills of blood and blood products by following recommended precautions from the Centers for Disease Control (CDC). Always wear gloves when doing so.

Nursing responses to control infection at the resident level

1. Know your residents well and report any abnormal changes in behavior or symptoms.
2. Provide nursing measures using optimum technique, following the principle of cleaning from clean to dirty.
3. Residents on antibiotics may receive too much and side infections can occur. Report these immediately.
4. Work to prevent decubiti from occurring; use stringent nursing measures to prevent infection and transmission of infection and skin breakdown.
5. Do not share articles of care between residents.
6. Work toward maintaining the activity and nutrition of residents.
7. Follow universal precautions, using gloves for contact with residents when doing mouth care, perineal care, skin care, and other procedures involving body fluids.
8. Wear masks, gloves, goggles, and gowns when assisting with care when the resident might cough or spray the contents of mucus discharge.

RULES TO FOLLOW: HANDWASHING

- Handwashing must be done before and after each nursing task, before and after direct patient contact, and after handling any of a patient's belongings.
- The water faucet is always considered contaminated. This means there are germs on it. This is why you use paper towels to turn the faucet on and off (Figure 7.4).
- If your hands accidentally touch the inside of the sink, start over. Do the whole procedure again.

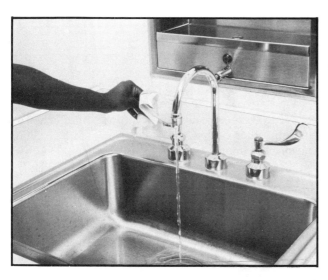

Figure 7.4.

- Take soap from a dispenser, if possible, rather than using bar soap. Bar soap accumulates pools of soapy water in the soap dish, which is then considered contaminated.
- Handwashing is effective only when:
  1. You use enough soap to produce lots of lather (Figure 7.5).
  2. You rub skin against skin to create friction, which helps to eliminate microorganisms.
  3. You rinse from the clean to the dirty parts of your hands. Rinse with running water from 2 inches above the wrists to the hands and then to the fingertips.
- Hold your hands lower than your elbows while washing. This is to prevent germs from contaminating your arms. Holding your hands down prevents backflow over unwashed skin.
- Add water to the soap while washing. This keeps the soap from becoming too dry.
- Never use the patient's soap for yourself.
- Rinse well. Soap left on the skin causes drying and can cause skin irritation (Figure 7.6).

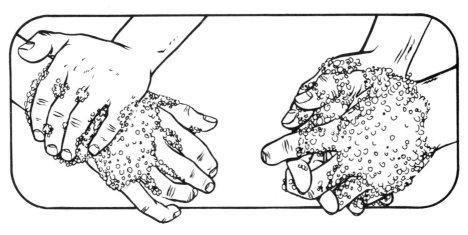

Figure 7.5.

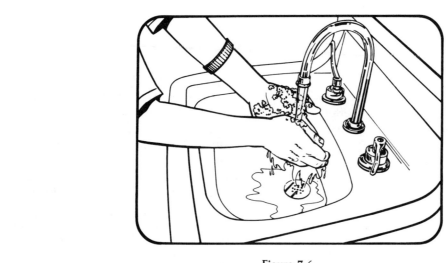

Figure 7.6.

ACQUIRED HUMAN IMMUNODEFICIENCY VIRUS

Human immunodeficiency virus (HIV), the virus that causes acquired immunodeficiency syndrome (AIDS), is transmitted through sexual contact and exposure to infected blood or blood components and perinatally (at time of birth) from mother to newborn. HIV has been isolated from blood, semen, vaginal secretions, saliva, tears, breast milk, cerebrospinal fluid, amniotic fluid, and urine and is likely to be isolated from other body fluids, secretions, and excretions. However, epidemiologic evidence has implicated only blood, semen, vaginal secretions, and possibly breast milk in transmission."[*] This quotation is taken from a publication produced by the Centers for Disease Control in Atlanta, Georgia. The publication continues to say that HIV is increasing in our population. Therefore, health care workers can be exposed to patients (residents/clients) who may be infected and cause exposure to the virus, especially when blood and body fluid precautions are not followed. The need for health care workers to consider *all* patients as potentially infected and to follow universal precautions to prevent exposure is emphasized.

The geriatric nursing assistant must know of the precautions and institute the procedures and policies of the health care setting where employed. The recommended universal precautions should be part of your health care setting and procedures. They have been reprinted for you in this book so that you can practice them and carry them out on the job.

Universal Precautions to Prevent HIV Transmission[†]

1. All health care workers should routinely use appropriate barrier precautions to prevent skin and mucous membrane exposure when contact with blood or other body fluids of any patient is anticipated. Gloves should be worn for touching blood and body fluids, mucous membranes, or nonintact skin of all patients, for handling items or surfaces soiled with blood or body

[*]From Centers for Disease Control, *Morbidity and Mortality Weekly Report*, August 21, 1987, Vol. 36, No. 25, p. 35.

[†]From Centers for Disease control, *Morbidity and Mortality Weekly Report*, August 21, 1987, Vol. 36, No. 25, p. 63.

fluids, and for performing venipuncture and other vascular access procedures. Gloves should be changed after contact with each patient. Masks and protective eyewear or face shields should be worn during procedures that are likely to generate droplets of blood or other body fluids to prevent exposure of mucous membranes of the mouth, nose, and eyes. Gowns or aprons should be worn during procedures that are likely to generate splashes of blood or other body fluids.

2. Hands and other skin surfaces should be washed immediately and thoroughly if contaminated with blood or other body fluids. Hands should be washed immediately after gloves are removed.

3. All health care workers should take precautions to prevent injuries caused by needles, scalpels, and other sharp instruments or devices during procedures; when cleaning used instruments; during disposal of used needles; and when handling sharp instruments after procedures. To prevent needlestick injuries, needles should not be recapped, purposely bent or broken by hand, removed from disposable syringes, or otherwise manipulated by hand. After they are used, disposable syringes and needles, scalpel blades, and other sharp items should be placed in puncture-resistant containers for disposal; the puncture-resistant containers should be located as close as practical to the use area. Large-bore reusable needles should be placed in a puncture-resistant container for transport to the reprocessing area.

4. Although saliva has not been implicated in HIV transmission, to minimize the need for emergency mouth-to-mouth resuscitation, mouthpieces, resuscitation bags, or other ventilation devices should be available for use in areas in which the need for resuscitation is predictable.

5. Health care workers who have exudative lesions or weeping dermatitis should refrain from all direct patient care and from handling patient care equipment until the condition resolves.

6. Pregnant health care workers are not known to be at greater risk of contracting HIV infection than health care workers who are not pregnant; however, if a health care worker develops HIV infection during pregnancy, the infant is at risk of infection resulting from perinatal transmission. Because of this risk, pregnant health care workers should be especially familiar with and adhere strictly to precautions to minimize the risk of HIV transmission.

Implementation of universal blood and body-fluid precautions for *all* patients eliminated the need for use of the isolation category of "Blood and Body Fluid Precautions" previously recommended by CDC for patients known or suspected to be infected with blood-borne pathogens. Isolation precautions [e.g., enteric, AFB (acid fast bacillus, the organism that causes tuberculosis)] should be used as necessary if associated conditions, such as infectious diarrhea or tuberculosis, are diagnosed or suspected.

CHECKLIST FOR HANDWASHING TECHNIQUES

Equipment: Soap, brush, paper towels, warm water

	Yes	*No*
1. Turn on water and adjust the temperature.	—	—
2. Wet hands with fingertips pointed downward.	—	—

	Yes	*No*
3. Apply soap to hands and wrists (using enough to produce a lather).	—	—
4. Rub hands in a circular motion, washing fingers by interlacing back and forth between each other. (Add water when necessary to keep moist.)	—	—
5. Use a nail brush if necessary. If none is available, rub fingernails on the palms of hands.	—	—
6. Rinse hands from the wrist to the fingers with fingertips pointed downward.	—	—
7. Dry hands with a paper towel.	—	—
8. Turn off faucet with the paper towel. (The faucet is always considered dirty.)	—	—
9. Throw the paper towel into the wastebasket.	—	—
10. Leave the area clean and neat.	—	—

Note: Jewelry should not be worn. Check on the policies of your facility.

CHECKLIST FOR DONNING AND REMOVING AN ISOLATION GOWN

Donning (Figure 7.7)

	Yes	*No*
1. Wash hands, roll up sleeves if wearing any sleeves.	—	—
2. Unfold gown so that opening is at the back.	—	—
3. Put arms into sleeves of gown and pull up over hands.	—	—
4. Tighten gown close around the neck and around uniform, making sure that uniform is covered completely.	—	—
5. Tie neck tie or fasten appropriately. (*Note:* Neck band and ties are always considered clean.)	—	—
6. Grasp ties on front and bring to back.	—	—
7. Grasp edges of back and pull together, making sure they cover uniform.	—	—
8. Tie waist ties. (*Note:* Waist ties are contaminated after being in unit.)	—	—

Removing

	Yes	*No*
1. Untie the waist ties.	—	—
2. If not wearing gloves:		
a. Wash hands and dry with paper towel.	—	—
b. Turn off faucet with dry paper towel.	—	—
3. If wearing gloves, remove and discard in trash container in room.	—	—
4. Wash hands using dry paper towel to dry hands. Use dry paper towel to turn off faucet.	—	—

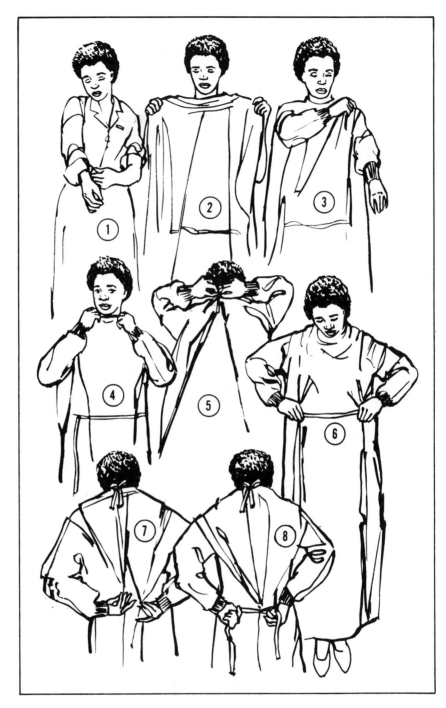

Figure 7.7. Gowning procedure.

5. Untie ties at the neck and reach inside neck band with both hands, pulling gown from inside away from you. Roll gown into a ball, inside out, as you take gown off.   —   —

6. Dispose of paper gowns in trash, linen gowns in hamper (Figure 7.8).   —   —

7. Remove mask. (*Note:* Ties on mask are always considered clean.) Dispose accordingly, depending on whether mask is disposable or linen.   —   —

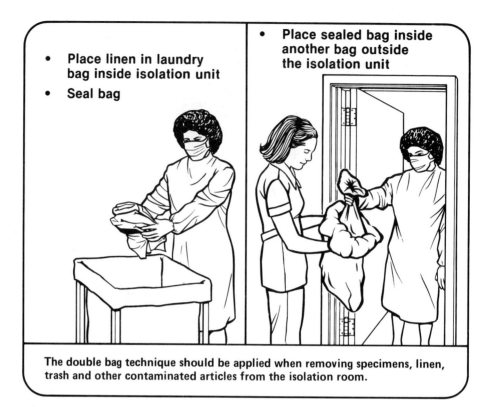

- Place linen in laundry bag inside isolation unit
- Seal bag

- Place sealed bag inside another bag outside the isolation unit

The double bag technique should be applied when removing specimens, linen, trash and other contaminated articles from the isolation room.

Figure 7.8.

	Yes	*No*
8. Wash hands using a dry paper towel to turn off faucet and a different dry paper towel to dry hands.	—	—
9. Open door with paper towel. Dispose of towel in unit before leaving.	—	—
10. Wash hands.	—	—

CHECKLIST FOR DONNING AND REMOVING MASKS

Donning (Figure 7.9)

	Yes	*No*
1. Wash hands.	—	—
2. Pick up clean mask and unfold if necessary.	—	—
3. Place mask over nose and mouth.	—	—
4. Tie top and then lower strings behind head.	—	—

Removing

	Yes	*No*
1. If wearing gloves, remove gloves first and then wash hands. (See checklist for gloving.)	—	—
2. Untie strings of mask in back of head.	—	—
3. Remove mask by holding strings and discard.	—	—

Note: If wearing gown, gown can be removed first, wash hands, and then proceed with removing mask.

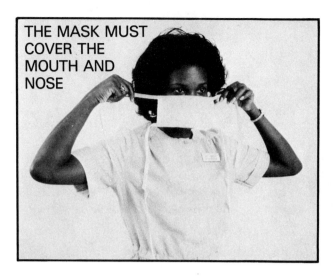

Figure 7.9.

CHECKLIST FOR DONNING AND REMOVING GLOVES

	Yes	*No*
1. Put on clean gloves. (If wearing gown, be sure cuff of gloves overlaps cuff of gown.)	—	—
2. When removing gloves (Figure 7.10), use preferred hand to pull off opposite glove *without* touching inside of opposite gloves. Discard glove.	—	—
3. Remove second glove by reaching inside the glove with ungloved hand and pull glove off. Discard glove.	—	—
4. Wash hands.	—	—

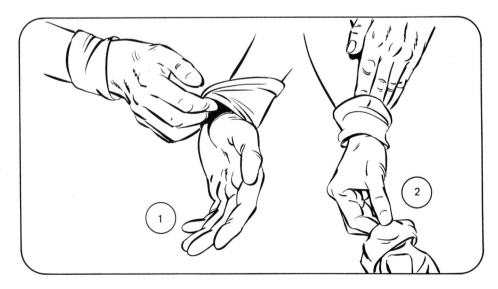

Figure 7.10. Removing gloves.

KEY POINTS

1. Geriatric nursing assistants are in prime position to apply infection control measures.
2. Geriatric nursing assistants should be able to use the terminology of infection control appropriately.
3. Handwashing remains the most important measure to be taken in helping to control infections.
4. The geriatric nursing assistant must be able to apply infection control measures to prevent any possibility of transferring the HIV virus.
5. Elderly people are very susceptible to infections because of age-related changes and decrease in efficiency of body systems.

SELF-CHECK

1. Make a list of 10 specific responsibilities that geriatric nursing assistants have in infection control.

2. Describe the difference between medical asepsis and surgical asepsis.

3. Mrs. White developed a bladder infection after a catheter was inserted. Is this a nosocomial infection? Explain.

4. Mr. Jones was admitted to the nursing home from St. Mary's Hospital. He had a decubitus ulcer on his sacral area which drains through to the bandages that cover the ulcer. Make a list of the precautions that need to be taken when caring for him.

5. The registered nurse is caring for Mrs. Asher today because she's receiving a pint of blood intravenously. You are asked to check on her every half-hour to be sure that she is comfortable. You notice some blood on the bed-side table and on the bed linen—it probably dripped there when the blood was added to the IV. What precautions will need to be taken?

6. Explain the statement: Infection control is everyone's business.

7. You are taking care of Mr. Bennett, who is coughing up mucus and sometimes needs to be suctioned by the charge nurse. Are any of the universal precautions needed when caring for him? If so, what are they, and why?

SUGGESTED ACTIVITIES

1. Attend community educational sessions that provide information on the acquired immune deficiency syndrome.
2. Read the labels on the disinfectants used in your facility to see how they help in aseptic measures.
3. Ask your charge nurse about which residents have infections and how they occurred. Find out what aseptic practices apply and if some practices were not followed.
4. Observe handwashing technique where you work. Report to the class the differences you see from what is recommended.

CLINICAL APPLICATION

Using the checklists in this unit, practice handwashing, and donning and removing masks, gloves, and gowns. Apply those techniques when necessary on the job. Check your facility's policies and procedures for any differences.

Accident Prevention

TERMINAL PERFORMANCE OBJECTIVE

Given information related to accidents of elderly people, be able to assist in prevention and apply skills that will lessen injury if a resident falls.

Enabling Objectives

1. Explain why accidents involving elderly people are usually serious.
2. List five reasons why elderly people are more prone to have accidents.
3. Explain the geriatric nursing assistant's responsibilities if he or she witnesses or is part of a resident's accident.

4. Make a list of actions the geriatric nursing assistant can do to help prevent accidents.
5. Describe what the geriatric nursing assistant can do to help avoid injury when assisting a resident while ambulating.

REVIEW SECTION

The geriatric nursing assistant should review with the instructor the age-related changes that may lead to accidents.

PREVENTING ACCIDENTS

Preventing accidents becomes very important to the elderly person for several reasons. A person with a severe injury may spend many days in rehabilitation and is exposed to a variety of complications. Independence may be lost because of the inability to function without assistance. Rehabilitation and a long recovery period are costly and stressful. The injury may be severe enough to cause death. Therefore, the geriatric nursing assistant must adopt an attitude of prevention and be conscious of conditions that may lead to accidents.

FALLS OF RESIDENTS

Falls constitute the greatest number of accidents of the older population. Often even minor falls cause the older person to be bedridden for a few days. The more bedridden the older person, the more complications.

Factors contributing to falls include the aging changes of decreased muscle strength, changes of center of gravity and posture, decreased sensory perception, impaired balance, confusion, antihypertensive drugs (and other drugs), and distractions that occur. Chronic disease conditions also contribute to falls.

Drop attacks have been identified as another explanation for falls. These are falls due to no well-defined reason other than a sudden loss of tone in the legs that causes an immediate fall. Environmental causes of falls have been identified: inadequate lighting, slippery surfaces, obstructions in hallways, and cords and other objects which are hard to distinguish from floor coverings.

Nurses who cannot prevent falls need to teach residents how to fall to prevent injury. Nurses should not blame residents for the falls; many are not preventable. Nurses can also warn residents who are considered high risk for falls to seek assistance for ambulation.

Another measure that nursing assistants can take is to monitor the areas to prevent obstructions and to become more aware of when falls are most likely to occur in order to try to prevent them. Monitoring of incident reports to see when most accidents occur will be of some help. Figure 7.11 shows a sample of a form that can be used to monitor the names and number of residents who appear to be high risk. This type of form can be used for monitoring residents who fall frequently. This information can be used to establish a plan of prevention. Take it upon yourself to develop a list of residents under your care who are prone to falls and see what you can do to help prevent the next fall.

The following checklists are provided for ambulating with residents. Some facilities require all residents who need assistance to be wearing gait (transfer)

PATIENT INCIDENT LOG

Patient's Name	Date	Time	Exact Location	Type of Incident	Type of Injury	Hospital Involvement	Environmental Problems

Figure 7.11. Patient incident log.

belts (Figure 7.12). These belts are an added device for supporting a person who may begin to fall. They also serve to provide reassurance to the care giver who assists a resident from a sitting position to a standing position.

CHECKLIST FOR AMBULATING RESIDENT WITH AND WITHOUT GAIT BELT

With Gait Belt

	Yes	No
1. Explain the procedure to resident.	—	—
2. Have resident properly dressed (in privacy) in slippers, robe, and so on.	—	—
3. Place gait belt on resident, explaining its use, pulling snugly in place.	—	—
4. Have the resident sit before walking; check pulse rate.	—	—
5. Monitor resident's condition (color, perspiration, feelings, strength).	—	—
6. Have resident stand; place your nearest arm around resident's waist, grasping gait belt.	—	—
7. Walk to resident's side, slightly behind resident. Encourage good posture.	—	—
8. Know walking distance, provide for rest stop; check pulse and monitor condition.	—	—

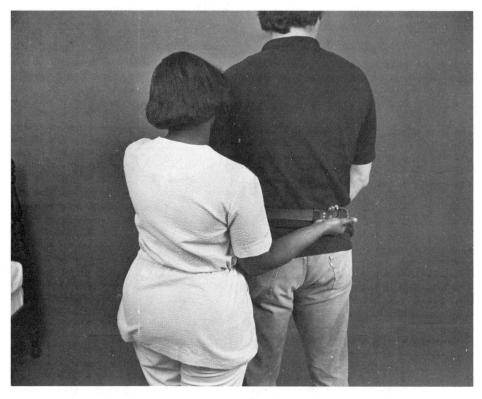

Figure 7.12. Ambulation with a gait belt.

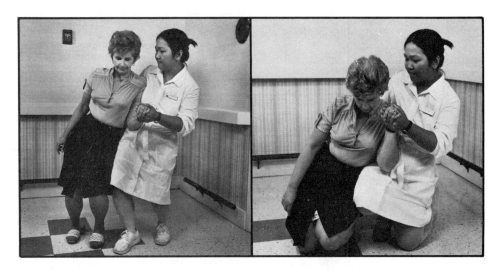

Figure 7.13. Easing the resident to the floor.

	Yes	*No*
9. Be sure that walking area has few distractions, is uncluttered.	—	—
10. Report any unusual reactions.	—	—

Without Gait Belt

	Yes	*No*
1. Repeat steps 1, 2, 4, 5, and 6 in procedure for ambulation with gait belt.	—	—
2. Walk at resident's side.	—	—
3. Place arm around waist if needed.	—	—

CHECKLIST TO PREVENT INJURY IF A RESIDENT FALLS

	Yes	*No*
1. Keep your feet apart, back straight.	—	—
2. Pull resident close to you, grab under arms, around waist, grasp gait belt if in place.	—	—
3. Gently lower resident and self, bend your knees, keep back straight (Figure 7.13).	—	—
4. Drop gently to floor.	—	—
5. Have resident checked by supervisor and/or M.D. before moving.	—	—
6. Obtain assistance to move resident back to bed.	—	—
7. Complete incident report; follow facility policies.	—	—

INCIDENT REPORTS

Whenever a resident falls, the care giver is required to write an incident report so that there is written evidence and a means of following up the incident. An example of an incident form is shown in Figure 7.14. When writing an incident

---

MEMORIAL HOSPITAL
ACCIDENT/INCIDENT REPORT

1. Patient ☒   Visitor ☐   Employee ☐   Other ☐

2. Date of this report <u>12/25</u> 19<u>xx</u>   Date of incident   <u>12/25/xx</u>

3. Name <u>Johnson, Henry A.</u>   Age <u>43</u>   Sex <u>Male</u>   Marital Status _____
   Department _____   Position _____

4. Location incident occurred at <u>Room 407</u>   Time <u>1:00</u> a.m.
          p.m.

5. Reported to _____ Patient seen by Dr. <u>Ralph A. Jones</u>
   _____ Time ___ a.m. _____ Time <u>1:05</u> a.m.
        p.m.   p.m.

6. Statement of doctor or resident (diagnosis, parts of body affected and treatment)
        Patient examined—no injuries sustained—left elbow slightly
        abraded—Merthiolate applied.
   _____ Attending Physician _____ M.D.

7. Describe incident and how accident occurred. (Statement of nurse or person in charge.)
        Patient found on floor—stated he attempted to get out of bed, slipped off of footstool and fell to floor.
        One rubber tip missing from stool. Slight abrasion of left elbow. No hospital property damaged.
   Signed _____ Title _____

8. Witness's name <u>Fred R. Smith</u>   Address <u>33 Yale St., New Brunswick, N.J.</u>
   Witness's name _____   Address _____

9. Name of machine involved _____

10. Kind of work performed by machine _____

11. Part of machine causing injury _____

12. Any protective device on machine _____

13. Action taken to prevent recurrence _____
    _____ Signed _____ Title _____
           mo   day   yr

14. Did employee lose time?   Yes ☐   No ☐   If yes, give last day worked ☐ ☐ ☐
                      mo   day   yr   mo   day   yr
    If unable to resume work, give probable date of return ☐ ☐ ☐   if already returned ☐ ☐ ☐

15. If patient accident, signed _____ Date _____
         Ass't. Adm. Nursing Service

    Reported to administration on _____ at _____ a.m.   Signed _____ Adm.
                              p.m.

Department director must complete necessary information in duplicate. Duplicate must be forwarded immediately to chairman of the safety committee.

Reviewed by safety committee on _____ Signed _____ Chairman.

(FILL OUT IN DUPLICATE)

Figure 7.14.

report, the care giver describes the facts only. The report should be written as objectively as possible.

As a care giver, the geriatric nursing assistant can observe the resident for any after effects of the fall. Daily monitoring for any changes of accident victims will allow early reporting and prevention of further complications.

KEY POINTS

1. Elderly people who have accidents will have more difficulty recovering than a younger person will.
2. There are age-related changes that may cause elderly people to be high risks for accidents.

3. Geriatric nursing assistants can help to prevent accidents by providing assistance to high-risk people.
4. An incident report must be completed when an accident occurs. These reports may help to identify causes and ways to prevent accidents.
5. All residents who have accidents must be checked frequently to prevent complications.

The Use of Restraining Devices

TERMINAL PERFORMANCE OBJECTIVE

After reading the information on resident safety and the use of restraining devices, and given checklists for application of the restraints, be able to apply the safety restraints.

Enabling Objectives

1. Identify reasons for restraining devices.
2. Review rights of patients that pertain to restraining devices.
3. Practice application of restraining devices using the checklists provided.
4. Identify geriatric nursing assistant responses for person with restraining devices.

REVIEW SECTION

The geriatric nursing assistant should review with the instructor rights of patients that pertain to the use of restraining devices and some of the effects of leaving devices in place without giving the proper nursing attention.

REASONS FOR RESTRAINING DEVICES

The uppermost reason for using any restraining device is to provide safety for the person. The safety problem needs to be explained to the resident and the resident's family. It is very upsetting to a family member to see a loved one in a restraining device without knowing the reason for it. Both the individual and family member may perceive the device as a form of restriction and punishment.

Restraints should only be used with a doctor's order. Nursing staff are not free to place a restraining device on a person without an order indicating what type of safety restraint is needed. Restraints may be needed for the following reasons: to help maintain correct posture, to keep a person from climbing out of bed and falling, to help keep an arm with an IV from moving if the person

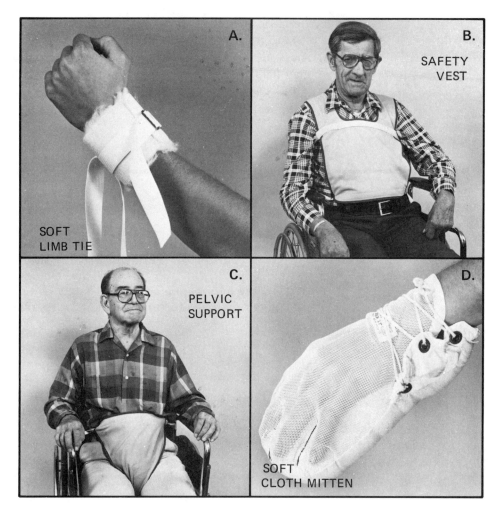

Figure 7.15. Soft protective devices.

is confused and swinging his or her arms, and to keep a mentally disturbed patient from causing harm to self and others (Figure 7.15).

Nursing responses for residents in restraints

1. Explain the use of the device to the person and person's family.
2. Apply in a calm manner.
3. Check the person at least every half-hour to be sure the device is not injuring the tissue or disturbing circulation. (Look for bruising of the skin, redness, and breaks in the skin.)
4. Temporarily remove the restraints according to the facility's policies (normally, every 2 hours).
5. Reposition the resident, check for any reddened areas of skin, and massage the area (when the restraints are removed).
6. Check on drinking fluids and toilet needs frequently, at least every 2 hours.
7. Plan to remove restraints as soon as the person's safety is determined.
8. Record as permitted all nursing measures given on the person's chart. Documentation of care of a person in restraining devices is usually required.

Under the Medicare law dealing with "Specified Rights," the federal government proclaimed the following on December 22, 1987:*

A skilled nursing facility must protect and promote the rights of each resident, including each of the following rights: . . . the right to be free from physical or mental abuse, corporal punishment, involuntary seclusion, and any physical or chemical restraints imposed for purposes of discipline or convenience and not required to treat the resident's medical symptoms. Restraints may only be imposed: (1) to ensure the physical safety of the resident or other residents and (2) only upon the written order of a physician that specifies the duration and circumstances under which the restraints are to be used (except in emergency circumstances specified by the Secretary) until such an order could reasonably be obtained. (Secretary in this instance refers to the Secretary of the federal government in Health and Human Services.)

It is very important to reassure the elderly person about the safety needs for restraining devices. The geriatric nursing assistant should convey a caring attitude and speak with sincerity about the need to protect the person from harm.

CHECKLIST FOR APPLYING LIMB RESTRAINTS

Equipment and supplies: Adjustable limb restraint(s)
   Note: Know the federal guidelines for application and removal of restraints.

	Yes	No
1. Check doctor's order or obtain authorization from immediate supervisor.	—	—
2. Assemble equipment.	—	—
3. Wash hands.	—	—
4. Identify resident. Explain procedure even if the resident is irrational or confused. (*Note:* In an emergency, restraints can be applied to prevent injury. The doctor is then contacted. The supervisor or authorized person makes the decision to apply restraints in emergencies.)	—	—
5. Place the soft edge of the restraint against the resident's skin. Wrap the restraint smoothly around the limb. Make sure that no wrinkles are present.	—	—
6. Pull both ends of the straps through the tab or ring on the restraint. Then pull the restraint secure, but not too tight, against the resident's skin. (*Caution:* If applied too tightly, the restraint could stop circulation or cause a pressure sore to form.)	—	—
7. Test for fit and comfort by inserting two fingers between the restraint and the resident's skin.	—	—
8. Position the arm or leg in a comfortable position. Limit movement only as much as necessary.	—	—
9. Secure the straps to the bedframe, stretcher frame, or other frame with a double-clove hitch. To make the		

*From *Congressional Record—House,* H 12989, December 22, 1987, Omnibus Budget Reconciliation Act of 1987, p. 196.

	Yes	*No*
double-clove hitch, bring the strap around the frame and then bring the strap up, over, and through the loop that has been made by the frame. Repeat the process for a double loop.	—	—
10. Recheck the resident before leaving. (*Caution:* Make sure the restraint is secure but not too tight.)	—	—
11. Observe all checkpoints before leaving the resident: Position resident in correct alignment, place call signal and supplies within reach of resident, lower bed to lowest level, elevate siderails, leave area neat and clean.	—	—
12. Recheck the resident frequently, at least every 30 minutes. Check color and temperature of skin. Remove restraint every 2 hours. Exercise the resident. Offer toileting and liquids; make bed and personal clothing changes as needed; give skin care to skin that is under the restraint.	—	—
13. Remove restraints when authorized by supervisor or physician. (*Note:* Restraints are removed when the physician or supervisor feels that the danger of self-injury by the resident has passed.)	—	—
14. Replace all equipment.	—	—
15. Wash hands.	—	—
16. Record the use and release of restraints, and all care in number 12 above, on the resident's chart according to facility policy. Report any unusual skin problems and emotional responses of the resident.	—	—

CHECKLIST FOR APPLYING A JACKET RESTRAINT

Equipment and supplies: Jacket restraint (sleeveless)
   Note: Know federal guidelines for application and removal of restraints.

	Yes	*No*
1. Check doctor's order or obtain authorization from immediate supervisor.	—	—
2. Assemble equipment.	—	—
3. Wash hands.	—	—
4. Identify resident. Explain procedure even if resident is irrational or confused.	—	—
5. Slip the sleeves of the jacket restraint onto the resident's arms. Usually, the solid area is on the front for the most security. However, it can be placed in the back.	—	—
6. Crisscross the straps in the back. Check all of the material to make sure that it is free from wrinkles.	—	—

	Yes	*No*

7. Bring the loose end of the strap through the hole in the jacket. The jacket should now completely encircle the patient. — —

8. Check the restraint to be sure that it is not too tight against the resident. (*Caution:* Excessive tightness could interfere with breathing.) — —

9. Position the resident in a comfortable position. Allow as much movement as possible without injury. — —

10. On each side of the bed or stretcher, do the following: Bring the straps down and secure on the frame with a double-clove hitch. — —

11. In a wheelchair, the straps can be attached to the back frame. (*Caution:* Never attach them to any part of the wheels.) — —

12. Recheck the resident before leaving. Check the resident's respirations. — —

13. Observe checkpoints before leaving resident: Position resident comfortably and in correct alignment, place call signal and supplies in reach, elevate siderails, lower bed to lowest level, leave area neat and clean. — —

14. Return to check the resident every 30 minutes. Check count and character of respirations, and color and temperature of the skin. Remove the restraint every 2 hours. Exercise the resident, offer toileting and liquids; make bed and personal clothing changes as necessary; give skin care to the skin under the restraint. — —

15. Remove the restraint when authorized by the supervisor or physician. (*Note:* Restraint is removed when the danger of self-injury has passed.) — —

16. Replace all equipment. — —

17. Wash hands. — —

18. Record the use and release of restraints and all care given in step 14, on the resident's chart according to the policy of the facility. Report any unusual skin problems or emotional problems. — —

KEY POINTS

1. Restraining devices are used for safety.
2. The geriatric nursing assistant must be very familiar with rights of residents in regard to the use of restraining devices.
3. There are nursing care measures for each person in a restraining device. Devices must be applied correctly and appropriate care given.
4. All restraining procedures are to be explained to the resident and the resident's family members or significant people concerned about the resident.

Assisting in Disaster Drill Procedures

TERMINAL PERFORMANCE OBJECTIVE

Given guidelines on fire drill and bomb threat procedures and safe carry and rescue techniques with procedure checklists, be able to perform the carry and rescue procedures and to participate in disaster drill procedures.

Enabling Objectives

1. Identify the main causes of fires in nursing homes.
2. Make a list of the steps to be taken when a fire occurs.
3. Identify where oxygen is stored in a nursing home and how it is secured.
4. Make a list of the precautions to be taken when oxygen is in use.
5. Describe the procedure to be taken if a bomb threat is made while you are on duty.
6. Practice the rescue procedures of the blanket pull and two-person carry.

REVIEW SECTION

The geriatric nursing assistant should review with the instructor the safety precautions in daily activities that help to prevent fires, how to respond to a fire and how to operate a fire extinguisher.

PROCEDURES IN THE CASE OF A FIRE

Fires in nursing homes have been known to reach national attention. Unfortunately, many lives have been lost, especially in the older nursing homes, where fire-preventive devices were not installed. Elderly people are vulnerable to such disasters because of their chronic disease conditions, slowed responses, and susceptibility to suffocation through smoke inhalation.

Fires in nursing homes may be intentionally or unintentionally started by residents. Fires have been started by residents who were angry and who wanted to commit suicide. Part of the nursing staff's responsibility is to be aware of residents with potential for starting fires (Figure 7.16).

Nursing homes are now inspected for fire-safe environments and devices that keep fires to a minimum. Good nursing homes will be equipped with a sprinkler system, smoke detectors, flame-retardant materials, fire drill procedures, routine fire drills, fire extinguishers strategically placed, fire doors, fire exit patterns, and continuing education of staff on rescue procedures in case of fire (Figure 7.17). Residents should wear bedclothes made of flame-retardant materials.

Rescue procedures and a fire drill procedure have been incorporated into this section. It is advisable for all geriatric nursing assistants to practice these procedures and to compare the fire drill procedure with the one used in the facility where employed. The basic parts of all procedures should be essentially the same.

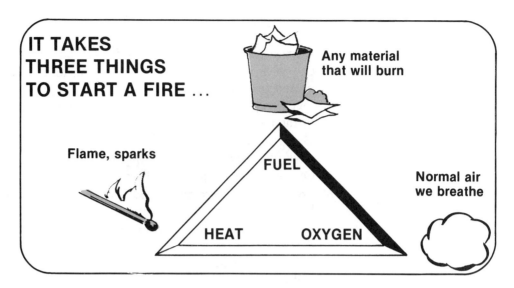

Figure 7.16.

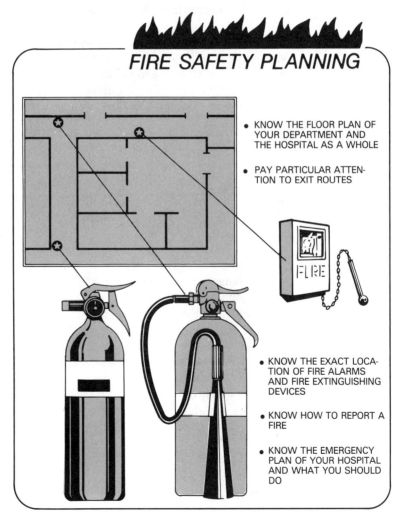

Figure 7.17.

Care of Oxygen Equipment*

1. Oxygen storage shall be provided in accordance with your facility fire code.
2. Oxygen cylinders shall be stored in areas with chains, sturdy portable carts, or approved stands.
3. Oxygen cylinders in use shall be on an approved cart or stand, not attached to the patient's bed.
4. Oxygen cylinders, unless in use attached to therapeutic equipment, shall have protective valve cap in place.
5. Oxygen cylinders shall not be stored in patients' rooms.
6. Tools used to serve oxygen equipment shall be kept clean and free from hydrocarbon material (grease, oil, etc.).
7. Smoking, open flames, and spark-producing devices are prohibited where oxygen is stored or administered.
8. All oxygen cylinders shall be tagged, indicating the amount of contents (e.g., half-full).
9. Warning signs shall be posted in areas where oxygen is administered.

General Description of the Fire Alarm System

Fire alarm boxes are located throughout the nursing home. These boxes are red with white handles and are fastened to the corridor walls. Any of these boxes may be used to turn in a fire alarm. If you discover a fire or see smoke anywhere in the nursing home, give the alarm. All employees must know the location of fire alarm boxes in their work areas and must know how to operate these alarms.

Chain of Command

The mechanics of firefighting are the responsibility of nursing home personnel only until the arrival of the local fire department. Upon their arrival, the senior officer of the fire department assumes control and direction of both firefighting and evacuation. They will conduct the firefighting procedure, designate safety zones, and issue instructions for movement or the evacuation of patients.

Until the fire department arrives, however, the supervising employee in the area of danger is in charge until relieved of this responsibility by his or her immediate supervisor or department head, the house supervisor, the assistant administrator, or the administrator.

General Instructions upon Discovering a Fire†

1. Remove any patient in immediate danger.
2. Give the alarm—use fire alarm box.
3. Begin taking first-aid firefighting measures.

*Printed with permission from Mrs. Jean Haezle, Administrator, Treasure Valley Manor Nursing Home, Boise, Idaho.

†Fire procedures are printed with permission from Mrs. Jean Haezle, Administrator, Treasure Valley Manor Nursing Home, Boise, Idaho.

Not one minute should be wasted between the discovery of smoke or fire and notification of the city fire department. Whenever possible, one employee should attend to the safety of endangered patients while another gives the alarm. Any employee who discovers or suspects a fire is authorized to give the alarm without securing permission from anyone at the time.

After removing patients in immediate danger and activating the alarm box, as an added assurance that the alarm has been transmitted, telephone the fire department, giving the exact location of the fire. Speak in a calm voice and be sure that the alarm operator has understood your message. Identify yourself and the location of the fire using the code "Signal F," not the word "fire" (e.g., This is Miss Jones—Signal F—Room 117).

Upon both directly turning in the alarm and notifying the fire department, begin taking first-aid firefighting measures.

If fire is in patient area

1. Move patients in immediate danger to safety. Be sure that alarm has been given.
2. Close all room, corridor, and stairway doors and windows.
3. Turn off all electrical and oxygen equipment except equipment necessary for safety of patients (determined by charge nurse).
4. Begin fighting the fire.
    a. Obtain proper extinguisher.
    b. Keep near door or avenue of escape.
    c. Aim extinguisher at base of fire.
    d. Stay low—out of heat and smoke.
    e. If fire gets large, get out of room or area, closing doors.
5. Ventilate only after fire is out.
6. If fire occurs at night, pull shades and turn on lights.
7. Don't panic! Don't shout "Fire!"

If fire is not in patient area

1. Be sure that alarm has been given. Close all room, corridor, and stairway doors in immediate area of fire. Gather ambulatory patients first. Appoint a person to act as guide and have all patients join hands and proceed to a safe zone. No patient must be left without guidance, for fear of panic.
2. *Wheelchair patients.* Use wheelchairs to take these patients to a safe place. Many will be able to walk with assistance. While some patients may be able to wheel themselves; they must never be left without guidance.
3. *Stretcher and helpless patients.* These patients cannot walk or otherwise fend for themselves. If movement to a safer portion of the same floor is possible, these patients must be wheeled in their bed, or wrapped in their bedding and dragged along the floor by pulling on the bedding, or a blanket can be used as a litter. Give each patient a wet towel to cover his or her face.

Admitting office: when an alarm sounds

1. Close doors of admitting office.
2. Send one person to front door to lead firefighter to fire in the event that the business office employee is busy.

If fire is in your area

1. Follow rules outlined in general instructions.
2. Make certain that patient register and all pertinent records and books are moved to safety.

Know the fire procedures, locations of fire alarm pull boxes, and how to operate fire extinguishers. This is your responsibility as a conscientious employee!

National Fire Protection Association Steps in Case of Fire

RACE is the acronym for the four steps to be taken when fire occurs. Many nursing home facilities follow these steps (Figure 7.18).

1. *R—Rescue.* Remove resident(s) from danger. Close the door to the room on fire.
2. *A—Alarm.* Pull the nearest alarm. Notify the fire department, giving exact location and type of fire, if known. Announce to all staff over the intercom using the facility's code (i.e., "F," "Code Red," etc.).
3. *C—Confine.* Close the doors to all residents' rooms and to the stairs, and all smoke doors. Evacuate residents near the fire.
4. *E—Extinguish.* Extinguish the fire with the extinguisher if it is small and can be confined.

The geriatric nursing assistant must know all four steps, and other staff need to know them as well so that you can all work together. Frequent fire drills are a necessity in order to be properly prepared if a real fire should occur.

Evacuation Procedures in Case of Fire

The following checklists provide the geriatric nursing assistant with the proper procedures for the blanket pull and the two-person carry.

SKILL CHECKLIST FOR SHORT DISTANCE RESCUE: BLANKET PULL (Figure 7.19)

Caution: Check with your facility about procedures to be used during times of emergency. In the event that a fire of major proportions occurs, and residents are in immediate danger, the following technique can be used. Be sure that the pull area is clear of sharp objects (see step 7).

	Yes	*No*
1. Position victim in supine position on floor.	—	—
2. Place blanket alongside victim so that it extends beyond feet and head. Fanfold two-thirds of the blanket next to victim.	—	—
3. Turn victim about one-eighth turn toward you, push blanket close to victim's back.	—	—

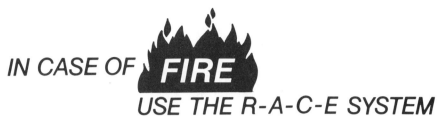

IN CASE OF **FIRE**
USE THE R-A-C-E SYSTEM

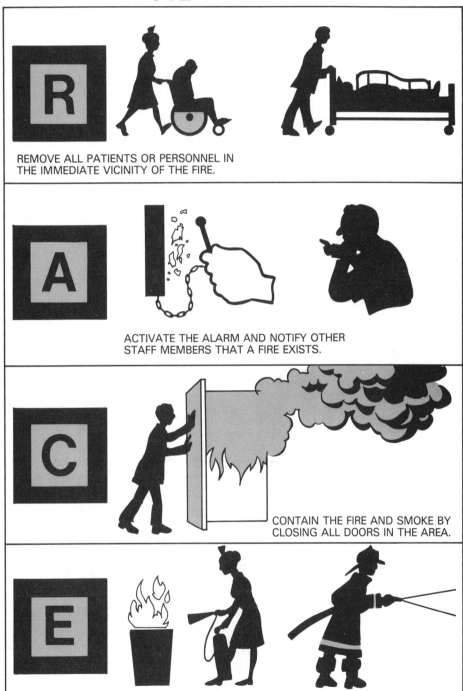

R REMOVE ALL PATIENTS OR PERSONNEL IN THE IMMEDIATE VICINITY OF THE FIRE.

A ACTIVATE THE ALARM AND NOTIFY OTHER STAFF MEMBERS THAT A FIRE EXISTS.

C CONTAIN THE FIRE AND SMOKE BY CLOSING ALL DOORS IN THE AREA.

E EXTINGUISH THE FIRE, IF IT IS A VERY SMALL FIRE, OR ALLOW THE FIRE DEPARTMENT TO EXTINGUISH IT.

Figure 7.18.

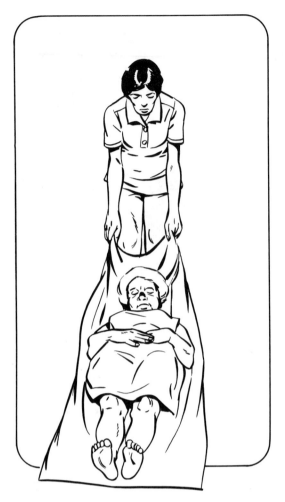

Figure 7.19. Blanket pull.

	Yes	No
4. Turn victim back over the folds of blanket. Pull through (one-third should be on opposite side, one-third under victim, and one-third nearest side).	—	—
5. Wrap blanket around victim, leaving face exposed.	—	—
6. Roll blanket in toward head from both sides, grasp roll in each hand, and pull victim as you move backward toward exit.	—	—
7. Area of pull should be cleared of any sharp objects.	—	—

CHECKLIST FOR TWO-PERSON CARRY (Figure 7.20)

The following carry can be used to transport a victim who has no head or back injuries. It is intended to move a person quickly to safety.

	Yes	No
1. Victim stands between two rescuers and places an arm across the shoulders of each rescuer.	—	—
2. Rescuers grasp each other's arm closest to victim.	—	—

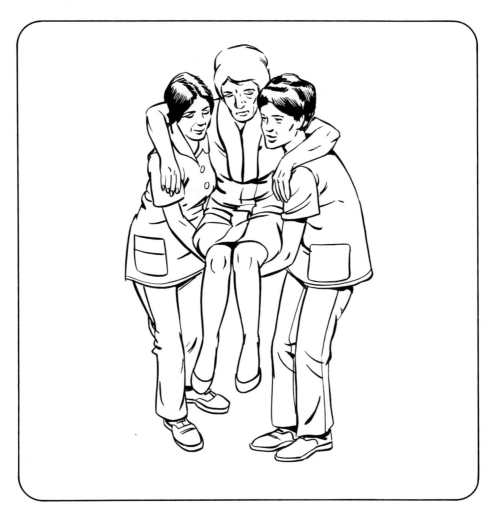

Figure 7.20. Two–person carry.

	Yes	No
3. Rescuers place grasped arms behind victim's knees and, on the count of three, pick up victim.	—	—
4. Rescuers' free arms support victim's back.	—	—
5. Victim is actually sitting on rescuers' grasped arms.	—	—
6. The rescuers can then walk together carrying victim.	—	—

PROCEDURES IN THE CASE OF A BOMB THREAT*

Upon notification of a bomb threat, the following procedure is suggested:

1. Fill out Bomb Threat Record as soon as possible (Figure 7.21).
2. Attract the attention of another employee if possible.
3. Call emergency number 911.
4. Call administrator.
5. Call director of nursing home if not in office.

*Printed with permission from Mrs. Jean Haezle, Administrator, Treasure Valley Manor Nursing Home, Boise, Idaho.

BOMB THREAT RECORD

Instructions: Be calm. Be courteous. Listen; do not interrupt the caller.

Time _____ Date _____

Caller's Identity:

Sex: ___ Male ___ Female ___ Adult ___ Juvenile Approximate Age ___

Origin of Call:

___ Local ___ Long Distance ___ Booth ___ Internal

Voice Characteristics		*Speech*	
___Loud	___Soft	___Fast	___Slow
___High pitch	___Deep	___Distinct	___Distorted
___Raspy	___Pleasant	___Stutter	___Nasal
___Intoxicated	___Other	___Slurred	___Lisp

Language		*Accent*	
___Excellent	___Good	___Local	___Not local
___Fair	___Poor	___Foreign	___Region
___Foul	___Other	___Race	

Manner		*Background Noises*	
___Calm	___Angry	___Factory machines	
___Rational	___Irrational	___Office machines	
___Coherent	___Incoherent	___Street traffic	
___Deliberate	___Emotional	___Party atmosphere	
___Righteous	___Laughing	___Bedlam	___Quiet
		___Music	___Voices
		___Mixed	___Animals
		___Trains	___Airplanes

Figure 7.21. Bomb threat.

Bomb Facts

Pretend difficulty when hearing. Keep caller talking if caller seems agreeable to further conversation. Ask questions like:

When will it go off? Time set _____

Time remaining _____

Where is it located? Building _____ Area _____

What kind of bomb? _____ Where are you now? _____

How do you know so much about the bomb? _____

What is your name and address? _____

If building is occupied, inform caller that detonation could cause injury or death.

Did caller appear familiar with plant or building by his description of the bomb location? Write out the message in its entirety and any other comments on a separate sheet of paper and attach to this checklist.

_____
Employee Signature

---

6. Charge nurses assign personnel to begin bomb search.
7. Follow instructions of person from police emergency.

Suggested Bomb Search Procedure*

1. Facility personnel will conduct the bomb search.
2. Do not arouse attention needlessly.
   a. Instruct visitors to leave quickly.
   b. Those visitors that are in patients' rooms should be instructed to close the door and to remain in the room until drill has been completed.
3. Initially, the following search will be made of the facility.
   a. This includes the following checks:
      (1) Checking the floor
      (2) Checking the walls
      (3) Checking the ceiling
   b. Do not look into every drawer, but do look in obvious places, such as trash containers.
   c. Place a notice on each door as it is searched.
   d. Go through every room in this manner.
4. After completion of above with nothing suspicious having been found, return to nursing station and report to charge nurse.

*Printed with permission from Mrs. Jean Haezle, Administrator, Treasure Valley Manor Nursing Home, Boise, Idaho.

    a. Begin a second search of entire facility. Be more thorough this time: look into closets, drawers, boxes, cupboards, washbasins, toilet tanks, windowsills, and so on.

    b. Mark doors a second time.

5. Charge nurse shall assign personnel to check all portions of the facility. This includes rest rooms, utility rooms, nursing stations, medicine rooms, foyers, coatracks, closets, unlocked closets, garbage cans, and so on.

6. Maintenance shall check areas thoroughly, especially those areas which, if destroyed, could render the facility inoperable. These areas include furnace rooms, main electrical switches and fuses, and outside store rooms. These should be kept in mind as possible danger areas.

7. Administration shall check offices.

8. Kitchen personnel shall check all incoming groceries and supplies, storage rooms, pantries, refrigerators, ovens, and stoves. These should be kept in mind as possible ongoing danger areas.

9. After completion of the search of inside areas, personnel shall search exterior. The search outside shall begin on the ground level, checking shrubbery, windows, basement walls, and so on, progressing upward to include the roof.

10. Police emergency personnel will determine if building shall be evacuated.

11. If object is found, contact emergency police personnel immediately.

12. Do not touch object!

Suspected Bomb with No Prior Notification

1. Call 911 and report findings.

2. Follow law enforcement officer instructions.

3. Call administrator.

4. Initiate partial evacuation if necessary.

KEY POINTS

1. Disasters in nursing homes need to be prevented. Once a fire occurs, getting all residents out is a tremendous problem. Fires have caused many deaths in nursing homes.

2. Practice and drills keep employees current—teamwork is essential.

3. Remain calm—it saves lives.

4. Know your facility's policies and procedures for all disasters. It is everyone's responsibility.

SELF-CHECK

1. What are four major causes of fire in nursing homes?

2. What three elements are necessary for a fire to start?

3. Whose responsibility is it to prevent fire in a nursing home?

4. List five prevention precautions you can take in your daily activities with residents and co-workers.

5. List the RACE steps you are to take if you discover a fire in a resident's room.

6. If you had to rescue a resident who is in bed and could not walk, what is one way you could do it when it is too time consuming to get the bed out of the room? Describe.

7. You ran out of wheelchairs and you must quickly remove a resident who cannot walk well from a building with much smoke. How can you and another assistant carry the resident? Describe.

8. What first five steps are you to take if you answer the telephone and the caller is telling you there is a bomb in your nursing unit?

9. What are two major attitudes that all staff must have in case of disaster?

10. Make up a fire safety checklist that considers the resident's immediate environment, use of oxygen and electrical equipment, smoking habits, and ability to move quickly. Your list should have at least 15 points for consideration.

SUGGESTED ACTIVITIES

1. Invite speakers to the class: family members whose loved one had to be restrained; a fire marshal to talk about a fire that occurred in a nursing home; a member of the police department to talk about bomb threat procedures.
2. Visit a laboratory to see the organisms that grow that cause infection. Discuss the benefits of infection control measures.
3. Invite an infection control professional to speak on the problems in nursing homes.

CLINICAL APPLICATION

1. Practice the isolation procedures in class and follow the guidelines of your facility on the job.
2. Apply the rules for prevention of infection in your daily activities.
3. Using the problem-solving worksheet provided, select a resident with a nosocomial infection and complete study of that person by completing the worksheet. Share with your classmates.
4. Practice the rescue procedures in class and be ready to use them if the need arises on the job.

WORKSHEET

Study of a Resident with Nosocomial Infection

Resident: _____   Infection: _____
　　　　　(first name only)

1. What are the possible reasons for this infection?

2. Considering the reasons, what could the nursing staff have done to prevent the infection?

3. What is the treatment?

4. What are the geriatric nursing assistant responses to help the resident?

8 SAFE POSITIONING, TRANSFERRING, TRANSPORTING

TERMINAL PERFORMANCE OBJECTIVE

Given skill checklists for procedures in positioning, range of motion, transferring and transporting, a simulated resident, and necessary equipment, be able to provide proper positioning of residents while in bed; to perform range of motion; and to transfer and transport residents according to the checklists.

Enabling Objectives

1. Describe the positions of supine, prone, semisupine, semiprone, Fowler's, and Sim's.
2. Identify the key areas of the body that need protection against pressure and decubiti formation when positioning.
3. Identify the safety principles involved when using lifting devices and transferring to wheelchairs or other vehicles.
4. Discuss the importance of psychologically preparing the resident or any client for transferring from bed with a lifting device or to any vehicle.
5. Describe the benefits of range of motion (ROM).
6. Practice the skills of positioning, range of motion, transferring, and transporting given in this unit.

REVIEW SECTION

The geriatric nursing assistant should review with the instructor proper body mechanics, injuries that could and have occurred using improper body mechanics, the procedures for positioning, range of motion, and transferring and transporting residents. These procedures have been learned before but are repeated here to improve skills. Geriatric specialists have also recommended repetition because improvement is always needed.

SPECIAL CONSIDERATIONS FOR POSITIONING THE ELDERLY

It must be kept in mind that the older person confined to bed will be a candidate for problems in several body systems. Circulation is slowed; therefore, blood distribution to the skin will be less, creating the potential for pressure areas. Lack of mobility and exercise adds to decreased circulation but also contributes to joint and muscle stiffness and may lead to contractions of the extremities. The respiratory system will also be slowed. Lying in one position is conducive to congestion of the lung and the condition known as hypostatic pneumonia, a pneumonia caused by constantly lying in one position. The elderly person confined to bed has a tendency to develop many complications.

The geriatric nursing assistant can do a great deal for the person in bed by positioning correctly to avoid the complications mentioned. In addition, the nursing assistant needs to change the person's position at least every 2 hours. For the very thin person, the change in position should be every hour. It is also necessary to avoid placing the very thin person directly on his or her side. The semiprone or semisupine position will keep the pressure off the hip bone. The checklists for these positions are included in this unit.

Range of motion of all extremities will help to avoid muscle and joint stiffness and the possibility of contractures. Encourage bed patients to breathe deeply every hour, taking 10 deep breaths each time. Have the patient cough as deeply as possible, having them cough 10 times each hour. These measures will help to avoid lung congestion.

SPECIAL CONSIDERATIONS WHEN TRANSFERRING THE ELDERLY

When preparing to transfer residents (whether using a lift or not), it is essential that the resident be prepared in a psychological manner as well as in a physical manner. Especially when using a lift, the resident might be very fearful of falling. The best way to alleviate the fear is by explanation of the procedure before the transfer is started. Explain the steps that will be taken and then repeat the explanation before each step is taken. The resident will have better understand-

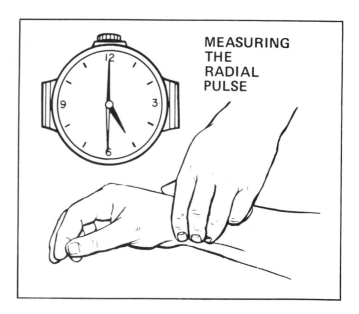

Figure 8.1.

ing and cooperate more willingly. Having the required number of people to help during the procedure will also give confidence to the resident that he or she is protected and will not fall. The geriatric nursing assistant needs to know the procedure well and have confidence in how to perform it. The confidence of the caregiver is reassuring to the resident.

Before transferring a resident, the geriatric nursing assistant should establish a baseline pulse by checking the resident's radial pulse (Figure 8.1). Knowing what the pulse is before transfer helps to evaluate the resident's tolerance of the transfer. A change in pulse from a moderate rate of about 60 to 70 per minute to 90 to 100 per minute may indicate that the resident is not tolerating the transfer. Other signs and symptoms to watch for include: perspiration, paleness of facial color, and complaints of dizziness and nausea. If these signs or symptoms occur, return the resident to bed and summon the nurse in charge.

CHECKLIST FOR POSITIONING IN THE SUPINE, PRONE, SEMISUPINE, SEMIPRONE, FOWLER'S, AND SIM'S POSITIONS

Supine Position

Resident is on his or her back.

	Yes	*No*
1. Head and neck are supported with small flat pillow that extends just below shoulders.	—	—
2. Arms, wrists, hands are at resident's side. Wrist is flexed. Handroll in place to prevent a closed fist. (Soft cone-shaped rolls may be used.)	—	—
3. Back is supported in lower back with small pillow as necessary.	—	—
4. Hips and upper legs are supported from below the waist to midthigh by towels, small rolled blanket, or trochanter roll.	—	—
5. Knees have support of small pillows or pads. Do not apply pressure directly behind the knee. Avoid using gatch on bed and overflexing the knee.	—	—
6. Heels are supported off the bed by small pillow or feet are extended over edge of mattress.	—	—
7. Toes have a footboard for support. Toes should be straight up.	—	—

Prone Position

Resident is lying on stomach.

1. Head and neck are supported with small flat pillow. Avoid large pillow.	—	—
2. Shoulders may need small pads to protect and give support if arms are at sides.	—	—
3. Arms, wrists, and hands are at a comfortable side position; usually arms are flexed at right angles. Hands may need handroll or cone to keep from a closed-fist action.	—	—

	Yes	*No*
4. Elbows have padding to keep pressure off area.	—	—
5. Abdomen has small flat pillow for support.	—	—
6. Hips and upper legs are supported by small pillow or rolled towels (trochanter roll); small pads are placed above and below knees to prevent additional pressure on the knees.	—	—
7. Feet are extended off mattress by use of pillow under lower legs. Allow resident to extend lower legs periodically to prevent any contracture from developing in joint.	—	—

Semisupine Position

Resident is halfway between back-lying and side-lying position (Figure 8.2).

	Yes	*No*
1. Head and neck are supported by regular-size pillow.	—	—
2. Shoulder and back are supported with rolled pillow.	—	—
3. Arms, wrists, and hands are comfortably supported by small pillow. Handrolls or cones are used to prevent a closed-fist action.	—	—
4. Both legs are extended with the bottom leg separated from the top leg by a pillow. The top leg is a little behind the bottom leg and resting on the pillow so that it is level with the hip joint.	—	—
5. Lower foot may need small pad to prevent pressure on the bed.	—	—

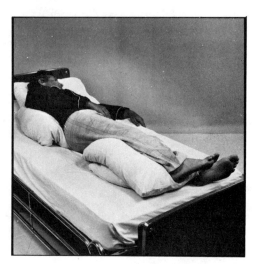

Figure 8.2. Semisupine position.

Semiprone Position

Resident is halfway prone and side-lying position (Figure 8.3).

	Yes	*No*
1. Head and neck are supported by regular pillow; head is turned to the side.	—	—
2. Arms, wrists, and hands are supported comfortably.		

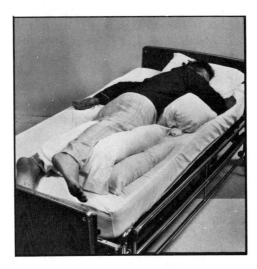

Figure 8.3. Semiprone positon.

Handrolls or cones are used as needed. Lower arm is
behind resident. Upper arm is partly supported by rolled
pillow under resident's chest.   —   —

3. Both legs are extended, lower leg and upper leg are supported by pillows.   —   —

4. Pillow under resident's chest and pillow under resident's
legs keep the resident from being flat on back or face
down in bed.   —   —

5. Small pads may be needed for any area that causes pressure on resident's feet.   —   —

6. Footboard should be in place.   —   —

Fowler's Position

Resident is in an upright position. See figure 8.4(a) and 8.4(b).

1. Head and neck are supported by regular pillow that extends just below shoulders. Head of bed is elevated.   —   —

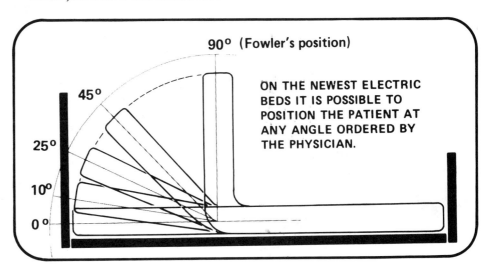

Figure 8.4(a). Fowler's position.

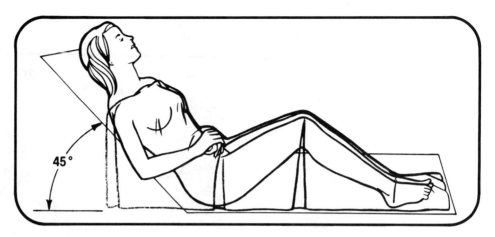

Figure 8.4(b).   Fowler's position.

	Yes	No
2. Arms are supported by pillows. Handroll in place as needed. Wrists are hyperextended with fingers and thumb higher than wrists.	—	—
3. Small pillow may be placed at lower back.	—	—
4. Small pads are placed under thighs and lower legs to give slight flexion to knees.	—	—
5. Lower foot may need small pad to prevent pressure from the bed.	—	—
6. Footboard should be in place.	—	—

Sim's Position

Resident is turned to either side (Figure 8.5); the left side is used for enema instillation.

1. Head and neck are supported with small pillow.   —   —
2. Resident's lower arm may extend behind. A small pillow may be used for support, but is not necessary for a short period of time, as in giving enemas. Upper arm rests on the bed. For a longer period of time, use small pillow for support.   —   —

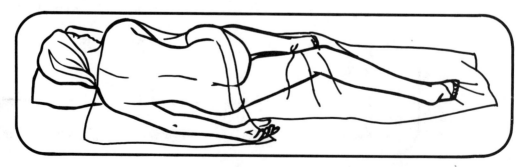

Figure 8.5.   Sim's position.

	Yes	*No*
3. Follow positioning of hand and wrists as for a longer period of time; for enemas, no additional measures are necessary.	—	—
4. Lower leg is extended, upper arm is flexed. For positioning other than enemas, place a pillow between the legs.	—	—
5. Use footboard for feet support; place padding under feet if using position for long periods of time.	—	—

CHECKLIST FOR RANGE-OF-MOTION EXERCISES

Equipment: Bath blanket

Note: Always support the joint you are exercising by placing one hand behind or under the joint.

	Yes	*No*
1. Wash your hands.	—	—
2. Identify the patient and explain procedure.	—	—
3. Provide privacy. Cover patient with bath blanket. Fanfold top linen to foot of bed.	—	—
4. Place the patient in a supine position with knees extended and arms at the side.	—	—
5. Lower the side rail on the near side of the bed.	—	—
6. Exercise the neck:		
Head flexion and extension. With patient's body straight, gently move head down, up and backward, then straighten neck again. See figure 8.6(a).	—	—
Right/left rotation. With head and body straight, gently rotate head to the right. Come back to starting position, then rotate head to the left. See figure 8.6(b).	—	—
Right/left lateral flexion. With body and head straight, move head gently toward the right shoulder. Come back		

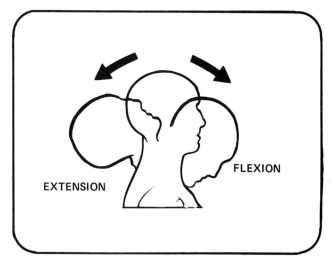

Figure 8.6(a).

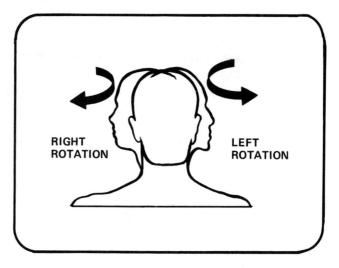

Figure 8.6(b).

	Yes	No

to starting position, then move head toward the left shoulder. Use the weight of the head to help move it. See figure 8.6(c).   ___   ___

7. Move to shoulder:
Shoulder flexion. With elbow straight, raise arm over head, then lower, keeping arm in front of you. See figure 8.6(d).   ___   ___

Shoulder abduction and adduction. With elbow straight, and supporting elbow and wrist, bring arm out to side and then return to side. See figure 8.6(e).   ___   ___

Shoulder internal and external rotation. Bring arm out to the side below shoulder level. Turn arm back and forth so forearm points down toward feet, then up toward head. With arm alongside body and elbow bent at 90 degrees, turn arm so forearm points across stomach, then out to side.   ___   ___

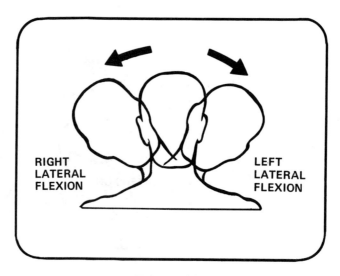

Figure 8.6(c).

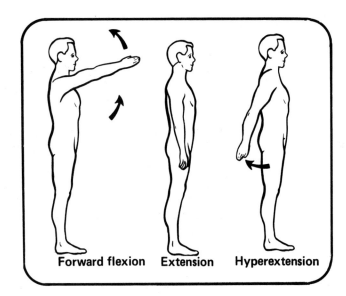

Figure 8.6(d).

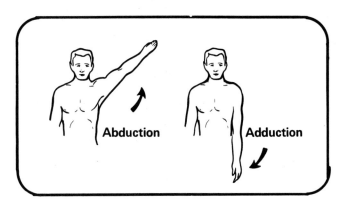

Figure 8.6(e).

	Yes	*No*
Shoulder horizontal adduction and abduction. Keep arm at shoulder level, reach across chest past opposite shoulder, then reach out to the side.	—	—
8. Exercise each elbow, wrist, and forearm:		
Elbow flexion and extension. With arm alongside body, bend elbow to touch shoulder, then straighten elbow out again. See figure 8.6(f).	—	—
Forearm pronation and supination. With arm alongside the body and elbow bent to 90 degrees, turn forearm so that palm faces toward head, then toward feet.	—	—
Wrist flexion and extension. Bend wrist up and down. See figure 8.6(g).	—	—
Ulnar and radial deviation. Bend wrist from side to side, keeping fingers together. See figure 8.6(h).	—	—
9. Exercise each finger:		
Finger flexion and extension. Make a fist, then straighten fingers out together. See figure 8.6(i).	—	—

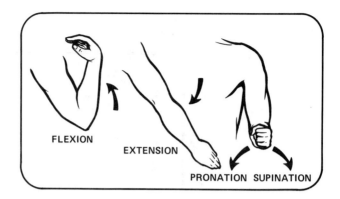

Figure 8.6(f).

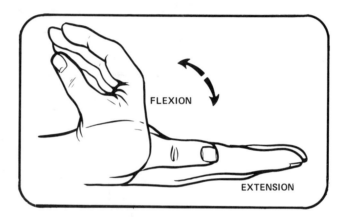

Figure 8.6(g).

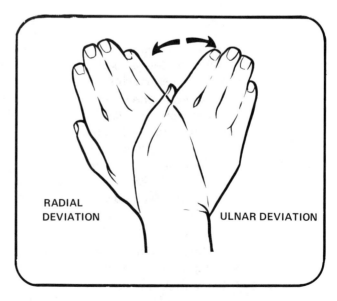

Figure 8.6(h).

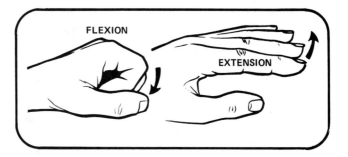

Figure 8.6(i).

	Yes	No

Individual finger flexion and extension. Move each joint individually. Touch tip of each finger to its base, then straighten each finger in turn.

Finger adduction and abduction. With fingers straight, squeeze fingers together, then spread them apart. See figure 8.6(j).

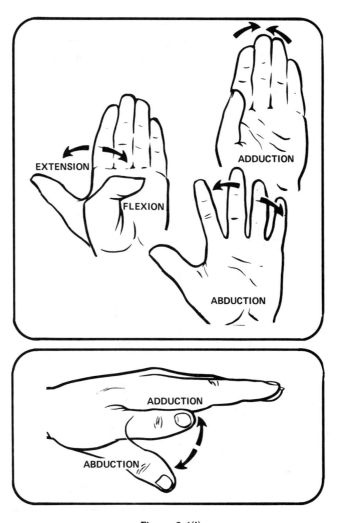

Figure 8.6(j).

	Yes	*No*

Finger/thumb opposition. Touch thumb to the tip of each finger to make a circle. Open hand fully between touching each finger.   —   —

10. Exercise each hip, knee, and ankle:
    Hip/knee flexion and extension. Keep areas not being exercised covered. (Be sure perineal area is covered.) Bend knee and bring it up toward chest, keeping foot off bed. Lower leg to bed, straightening knee as it goes down.   —   —

    Straight leg raising. Keeping the knee straight, raise leg up off the bed.   —   —

    Hip abduction and adduction. With leg flat on bed and knee kept pointing to ceiling, slide leg out to the side. Then slide it back to touch across the other leg. See figure 8.6(k).   —   —

    Hip internal and external rotation. With legs flat on bed and feet apart, turn both legs so that knees face outward. Then turn them in to face each other. See figure 8.6(l).   —   —

11. Exercise each foot:
    Ankle dorsiflexion and plantar flexion. Bend ankle up, down, and from side to side. See figure 8.6(m).   —   —

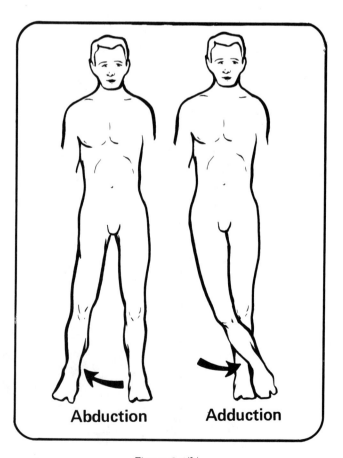

Abduction   **Adduction**

Figure 8.6(k).

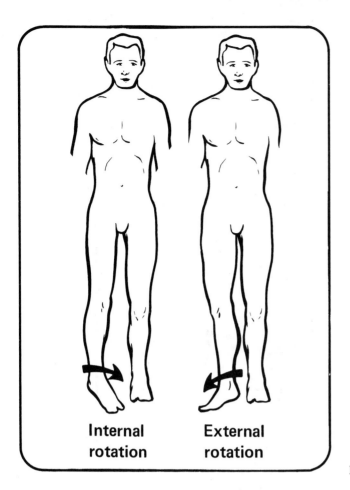

Internal
rotation

External
rotation

Figure 8.6(l).

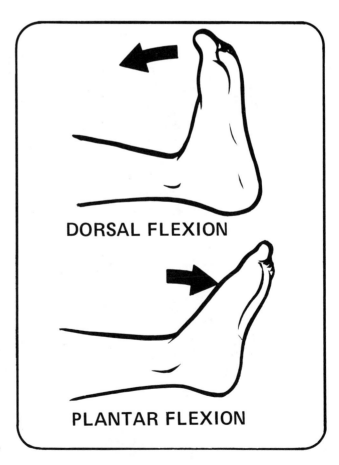

DORSAL FLEXION

PLANTAR FLEXION

Figure 8.6(m).

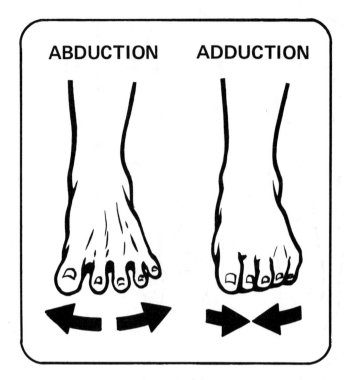

Figure 8.6(n).

	Yes	*No*
Toe flexion and extension. Bend and straighten each toe. See figure 8.6(n).	—	—
12. Make the resident comfortable. Cover with top sheets and remove bath blanket; place in dirty laundry.	—	—
13. Be sure the signal cord is within easy reach.	—	—
14. Raise the siderails.	—	—
15. Wash your hands.	—	—
16. Report and record the procedure and observations. Be sure to note patient's tolerance and progress with the exercises.	—	—

Note: Many of these motions can be done by care giver and resident when resident is bathing, dressing, or doing other daily activities.

TRANSFERRING A RESIDENT FROM PLACE TO PLACE

Mechanical Lifts (Hydraulic Lifts)

The hydraulic lift is used to transfer residents from bed to chair or chair to bed (Figure 8.7). It can usually be used for residents weighing up to 300 pounds. (Check with the policy of the facility.) The use of the lift is done with caution; two nurses are needed, one as a main operator, the second as a guide and overseer of the operation. A second person adds reassurance and support to the resident as well.

Mechanical lifts need to be checked routinely for good repair and operation. Some residents may become frightened with the move based on a mechanical

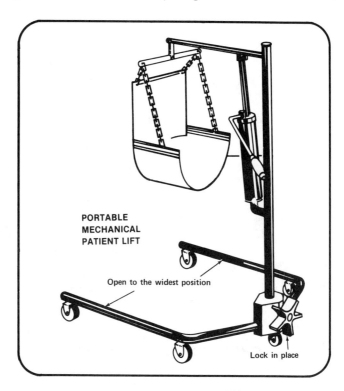

PORTABLE
MECHANICAL
PATIENT LIFT

Open to the widest position

Lock in place

Figure 8.7. Mechanical lift.

device. The nurses who help to transfer a resident must have confidence that they can operate the equipment safely. Practice using the equipment until you are very comfortable with it.

Lifts do vary in nursing homes. Follow the checklist provided in your facility. The checklist in this unit is very general and needs to be adapted to each different type of lift. However, some of the steps will always be the same.

CHECKLIST FOR TRANSPORTING A RESIDENT WITH A MECHANICAL LIFT*

	Yes	*No*
1. Assemble your equipment, check all parts for repair.	—	—
2. Wash your hands.	—	—
3. Explain procedure to resident, demonstrate how equipment works if this is the first time for the resident. Repeat explanation as you proceed.	—	—
4. Obtain a second nurse to help.	—	—
5. Provide privacy.	—	—
6. Provide confidence and reassurance as needed.	—	—
7. Lock wheels of bed. Lock wheels of lift.	—	—
8. Position lift at side of bed; open base to widest point. Move overhead bar over resident; place canvas seat under resident, or place pieces of lift to go under resident according to type of lift.	—	—

*Procedure modified and printed with permission of Idaho Veterans' Home, Boise, Idaho.

	Yes	No

9. Hook seat piece(s) to appropriate hooks, and hook up to overhead lift. *Make sure that sides are equal.*   —   —

10. Close the valve on the lift and gradually pump up the lift.   —   —

11. Second nurse uses hands to guide the lifting of the resident.   —   —

12. Lift resident off bed slightly. Check all connections. Slowly move the lift over the chair to receive resident. Second nurse guides the action and stays close to resident, giving support to the resident's feet. Guide resident into chair.   —   —

13. Remove hooks from the canvas seat carefully. Leave the canvas seat in place on chair under resident.   —   —

14. Arrange resident in alignment. Assure comfort.   —   —

15. Remove equipment until needed to transport resident back to bed. Wash hands.   —   —

CHECKLIST FOR TRANSFERRING A RESIDENT TO A WHEELCHAIR
(Figure 8.8a and b)

Equipment: Clean wheelchair with padding or protection; sheet or blanket for privacy and warmth to protect patient
   Note: Wash hands before procedure.

	Yes	No

1. Identify the patient and provide for privacy.   —   —

2. Explain the entire procedure and be sure that the patient understands when he or she will help. Reinforce

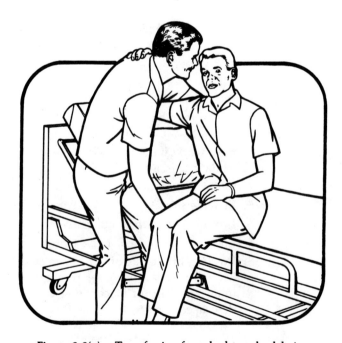

Figure 8.8(a).   Transferring from bed to wheelchair.

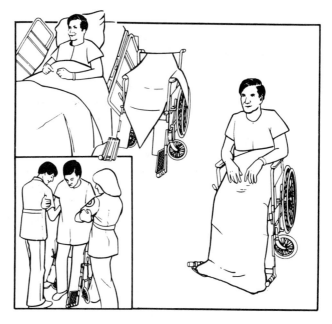

Figure 8.8(b). Two-person transfer from bed to wheelchair.

	Yes	No
directions as you perform the transfer. Check patient's pulse.	—	—
3. Adjust the bed height to the low position. You can raise the head of the bed so that the patient is sitting up. Be sure that the bed brakes are locked so that the bed does not move.	—	—
4. Bring the wheelchair up next to the side of the bed. If your patient is paralyzed or weak on one side, place the chair closest to the strong or unaffected side.	—	—
5. Lock the wheels on the chair. It may be helpful to have a second person hold the chair to be sure that it will not move or slide.	—	—
6. Fold the footrests completely up and out of the way.	—	—
7. Help the patient to move over in bed to within 5 or 6 inches of the edge of the bed.	—	—
8. Assist in putting on socks, shoes, and robe.	—	—
9. Assist the patient to swing his or her legs over the edge of the bed and sit up: Place one of your arms around the patient's shoulder and your other arm over and under the patient's knees. As you rotate your weight from your forward leg near the bed to your rear leg, swing the patient's shoulders up and legs off the bed. The patient should be sitting with his or her hips near the edge of the bed.	—	—
10. Give the patient time for the circulation to adjust to the upright position before your proceed with the transfer. Check resident's pulse and reinforce instructions during the procedure.	—	—

	Yes	*No*
11. Instruct resident to place hands on your shoulders. You place your hands and arms around the resident, under the axilla.	—	—
12. Explain what you want the resident to do. On the count of three, have the resident move to a standing position. You move in close to the resident.	—	—
13. Help the resident turn or pivot and move back until legs touch the wheelchair.	—	—
14. Have resident lower into wheelchair. You bend your knees and lower with resident, keeping back straight.	—	—
15. Assist resident to adjust into wheelchair. Check pulse for any distinct change. Assess tolerance to the move.	—	—
16. Cover resident as necessary and assist to move in wheelchair to place of choice.	—	—
17. Wash hands.	—	—

Note: Sometimes it is necessary to put padding in the seat of the wheelchair or to place a device to help prevent pressure. Pressure areas can develop if residents are in wheelchairs for longer than an hour. Residents should have a position change or readjustment of position at least every hour.

CHECKLIST FOR TRANSFERRING A RESIDENT FROM WHEELCHAIR TO BED

	Yes	*No*
1. The bed should be in the low position and locked.	—	—
2. Bring the wheelchair up next to the bed and lock the wheels.	—	—
3. Have the resident lift his or her feet and fold the footrests up and out of the way.	—	—
4. Have the resident place both hands on the arms of the chair. Help resident to stand using the same grasp procedure around the body under the axilla. Lower your body, bend knees. On count of three, have resident push up as you rise.	—	—
5. When standing, the resident should turn so that his or her back is to the bed.	—	—
6. Instruct the resident to sit on the edge of the bed and then work back on the bed until he or she is securely seated. Remove robe, shoes, and socks.	—	—
7. Assist the resident to lie down; swing the legs up onto the bed. Arrange the top bed linen comfortably and put up the siderail if needed.	—	—
8. Arrange personal articles within reach.	—	—
9. Assure alignment.	—	—
10. Place call button within reach.	—	—
11. Store wheelchair.	—	—
12. Wash hands.	—	—

Transporting in a Wheelchair

See Figure 8.9(a), (b), and (c).

1. Always explain where resident is going or ask where he or she wants to be.
2. Push wheelchair from behind, always aware of resident's position and safety.

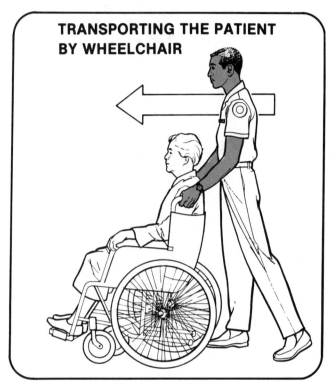

Figure 8.9(a). Transporting.

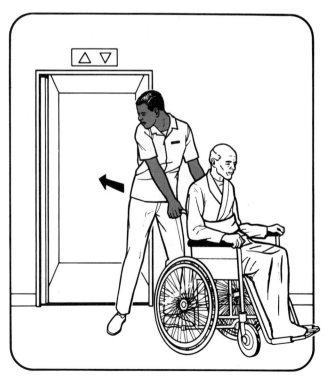

Figure 8.9(b). Transporting.

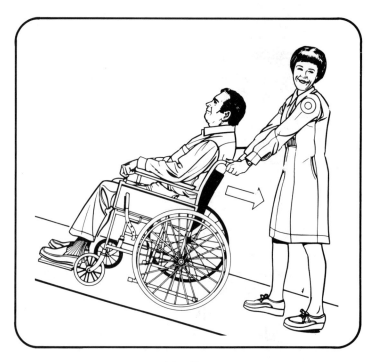

Figure 8.9(c).   Transporting.

3. When going in an elevator, turn wheelchair around so that resident goes in backward. (This protects resident from knocking into other people.)
4. When going down a ramp, turn wheelchair so that the resident is facing uphill. (This protects resident from falling forward as you go down the ramp. Your body keeps wheelchair from running out of control.)

Transferring to the Automobile

The geriatric nursing assistant will have the opportunity to transfer a person into and out of an automobile (Figure 8.10). As the nursing assistant works toward the rehabilitation of each resident, he or she will see some of them go on to more independent living. Residents who leave the nursing home will require some assistance in getting in and out of automobiles. The checklist provided to help you learn that skill can also be taught to family members who will take over that assistance.

CHECKLIST FOR TRANSFER OF RESIDENT IN AND OUT OF AN AUTOMOBILE*

Transfer into an Automobile

	Yes	*No*
1. Be sure that passenger seat (front seat) is as far back as possible.	—	—
2. Explain procedure to resident and give instructions throughout procedure.	—	—

*Printed with permission from Capital Care Center, Boise, Idaho.

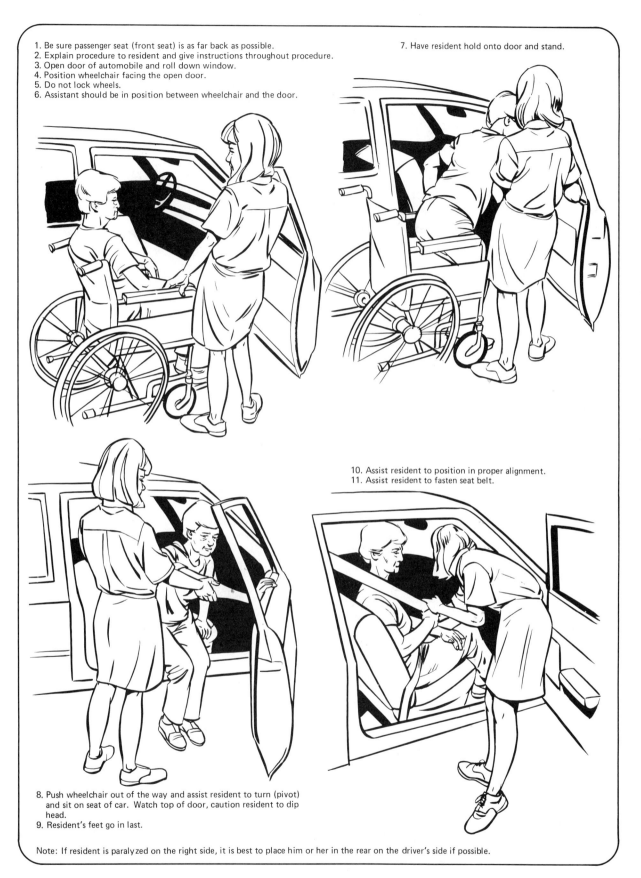

1. Be sure passenger seat (front seat) is as far back as possible.
2. Explain procedure to resident and give instructions throughout procedure.
3. Open door of automobile and roll down window.
4. Position wheelchair facing the open door.
5. Do not lock wheels.
6. Assistant should be in position between wheelchair and the door.

7. Have resident hold onto door and stand.

10. Assist resident to position in proper alignment.
11. Assist resident to fasten seat belt.

8. Push wheelchair out of the way and assist resident to turn (pivot) and sit on seat of car. Watch top of door, caution resident to dip head.
9. Resident's feet go in last.

Note: If resident is paralyzed on the right side, it is best to place him or her in the rear on the driver's side if possible.

Figure 8.10. Auto transfer.

	Yes	No
3. Open door of automobile and roll down window.	—	—
4. Position wheelchair facing the open door.	—	—
5. Do not lock wheels.	—	—
6. Assistant should be in position between wheelchair and door.	—	—
7. Have resident hold onto door and stand.	—	—
8. Push wheelchair out of the way and assist resident to turn (pivot) and sit on seat of car. Watch top of door, caution resident to dip head.	—	—
9. Resident's feet go in last.	—	—
10. Assist resident to position in proper alignment.	—	—
11. Assist resident to fasten seat belt.	—	—

Note: If resident is paralyzed on the right side, it is best to place him or her in the rear on the driver's side if possible.

Transfer out of Automobile to Wheelchair

	Yes	No
1. Open door of automobile, roll down window.	—	—
2. Explain procedure to resident and give instructions throughout procedure.	—	—
3. Assist resident to turn to doorway, place feet on the ground.	—	—
4. Position wheelchair facing door.	—	—
5. Leave wheelchair unlocked.	—	—
6. Have resident place one hand on back of car seat and one hand on the open door to assist to a standing position.	—	—
7. Assistant is in front of resident and helping resident to standing position. (Watch top of door, caution resident to dip head.)	—	—
8. Move chair up to resident. Lock wheels.	—	—
9. Assist resident to turn (pivot) and sit in wheelchair.	—	—

KEY POINTS

1. Frequent turning of residents confined to bed will help prevent decubiti.
2. Proper positioning and frequent range of motion prevent complications.
3. Check safety of all equipment used in transfers.
4. Prepare residents psychologically and physically before transfers. Establish confidence.
5. Establish a baseline of information about residents before transferring them. Notify head nurse immediately if signs or symptoms occur indicating an intolerance to a transfer.
6. Apply good body mechanics for yourself and your residents.
7. Transport residents with care, obeying the rules of transport to prevent accidents.

SELF-CHECK

1. Describe the safety factors involved in using a lifting device in transferring a person into a wheelchair.

2. List the rules of body mechanics involved with transferring residents.

3. Mrs. Jones is very fearful of being transferred into a wheelchair. She always stiffens up and seems to fight the procedure. What can you do?

4. You are to transport Mr. Green in a wheelchair, using the elevator, from the third floor to the first floor. Describe the rules you will follow for transporting him.

5. Mrs. Grissom is 85 years old and weighs 85 pounds. She has severe arthritis of the right knee and is confined to bed with a fever. Write a plan of care to follow to help prevent complications. Consider the body systems that can be affected by her immobility.

SUGGESTED ACTIVITIES

1. Observe body mechanics of co-workers as they transfer residents. Investigate any injuries of co-workers and how these occurred. Report to class.
2. Invite physical therapist to class to demonstrate his or her techniques of transfer. Discuss how to help residents become less fearful of transfers.
3. Talk with your charge nurse about residents with pressure areas/decubiti and how these occurred. Discuss the care plan and treatments involved.
4. Incorporate the procedures in this unit in your daily care of residents. Monitor any improvement. For example, encourage range of motion as much as possible for a person who rarely wants to help himself or herself bathe and dress. Watch for little signs of self-help.
5. Check the equipment used for lifting and transporting to assure safety. Report any defective equipment.

CLINICAL APPLICATION

Apply the procedures in this unit at your place of work. Select a resident confined to bed and monitor the care given by using the worksheet provided. After about 2 weeks, report back to the class on progress or lack of progress made in the improvement of the resident's condition.

WORKSHEET

Positioning and Transferring Procedures

Procedures used for a resident: (Circle those that apply) Mechanical Lift, Transfers to Wheelchair, Positioning in Bed, Range of Motion

Resident: _____   Condition/diagnosis: _____
            (first name only)

1. Describe resident in a few words: (Age, sex, personality, functional ability [what he/she can/cannot do]).

2. Describe how/when you perform the procedures you circled above.

3. Describe what you did to try to help the resident and to have the resident help himself or herself.

4. Describe what improvements or lack of improvement occurred after 2 weeks. Give reasons why.

9 NUTRITIONAL AND FLUID BALANCES

TERMINAL PERFORMANCE OBJECTIVE

Given the special nutritional and fluid needs of the elderly, and checklists for monitoring elderly residents with nutritional or fluid deficits, be able to apply nursing assistant responses to help residents improve; and be able to perform nursing procedures for conscious and unconscious residents with obstructed airways.

Enabling Objectives

1. Review the anatomy of the digestive system in Unit 2 and the corresponding age-related changes.
2. Define fluid balance and its importance for aging individuals.
3. List the six basic elements of good nutrition, their functions, and the kinds of food in which they are found.
4. Identify four ways in which fluids are eliminated from the body.
5. Describe at least two conditions that unbalance the fluids required by the elderly person.
6. Describe why confusion occurs in an elderly person with fluid/nutritional deficits.
7. Discuss five ways to make mealtime pleasant for residents.
8. Prepare a list of five factors to monitor when an elderly person is receiving feedings by tube and by vein.
9. Perform emergency procedures for relieving a choking resident who is conscious and becomes unconscious, and for a resident who is unconscious with an obstructed airway.

REVIEW SECTION

The geriatric nursing assistant should review with the instructor the basics of good nutrition, special diets, fluid intake, and feeding the helping and helpless resident.

MEETING THE CHANGES IN THE DIGESTIVE SYSTEM THAT AFFECT NUTRITION AND FLUID BALANCES IN THE ELDERLY

The basic nutritional requirements for older people are essentially the same as for younger people (Figure 9.1). The elderly require less food and consequently, fewer calories than do younger active people. Olympic athletes consume over 5000 calories a day; a young active teenager requires over 3000 calories a day. On the contrary, the older, less active male usually needs about 2200 calories and the female around 1800 calories a day.

The age-related changes seen in Unit 2 indicate there will be more digestive problems because of decreased enzyme activity and less tolerance for fatty foods. Common problems that occur are related to a shrinking in the mucosal lining of the stomach (less acid secretion) and a relaxation of the sphincter muscle around the esophagus. The relaxation of the esophageal sphincter may cause a regurgitation of stomach contents into the esophagus, causing "heartburn."

Other problems include constipation, due in part to less motility (peristalsis) of the intestinal tract and a diet low in fiber. Diverticular disease of the colon is common in older people, especially females. A diverticulum is a sac-like formation that occurs in a hollow organ such as the intestinal tract. See figure 9.2(a) & (b). Feces become trapped and cause complications. If untreated, the sac can rupture.

THE BASIC NUTRITIONAL REQUIREMENTS

Proteins make up the essential part of every body cell. Proteins are known as the body builders because they repair tissue and bone. They are found in animal meat, fish, poultry, and dairy products as well as nuts and beans.

Carbohydrates are the fast energy foods that give body heat. They are found in such foods as cereals, breads, potatoes, pastries, fruits, and starches like spaghetti.

Fats provide energy and body heat. The energy provided by fats is longer acting than that for carbohydrates. Fats are found in butter, cream, whole milk, meats, fish, and nuts.

Vitamins help to regulate the processes of the body, such as repair and growth of bones, vitamin D; coagulation of blood, vitamin K; strengthening of body cells and gums, vitamin C; protection from night blindness and promotion of healthy hair and skin, vitamin A; and promotion of a healthy nervous system, vitamin B complex. Vitamin A is found in yellow fruits and vegetables. Vitamin B complex is found in whole-grain products and dried vegetables. Vitamin C is found in citrus fruits and dark green vegetables. Vitamin D is found in milk and fish-liver oils. Vitamin K is found in green leafy vegetables and cauliflower.

Minerals such as calcium and phosphorus build bones and teeth. Calcium helps to regulate heart activity and blood clotting. Phosphorus is important to the nutrition of body cells, especially nerve tissue.

Water is essential to all body processes and cell functions. Water aids in carrying nutrients to body cells and in the elimination of wastes from these cells. The body requires that approximately 2 to 3 liters (2000 to 3000 cc) of fluid be consumed daily, depending on the individual's condition.

Fluid and the Elderly

Water is essential to the elderly person who is easily dehydrated for lack of sufficient amounts. An elderly person with an indwelling catheter should have up

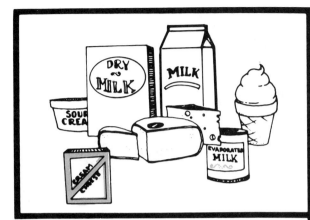

Group 1: Dairy Products

Milk

- 3 to 4 cups (Children)
- 4 or more cups (Teenagers)
- 2 or more cups (Adults)

Cheese, ice cream and other milk-made foods can be substituted for part of the milk requirement

Group 2: Vegetables and Fruit

- 4 or more servings

Include dark green or deep yellow vegetables; citrus fruit or tomatoes

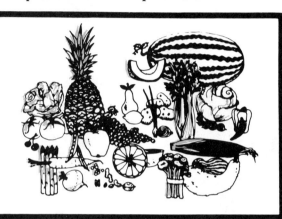

Group 3: Meat and Fish

- 3 servings

Meats, fish, poultry, eggs or cheese, with dry beans, peas, nuts as alternates

Group 4: Breads, Cereals, and Potatoes

- 4 or more servings

Enriched or whole grain. Added milk improves nutritional value

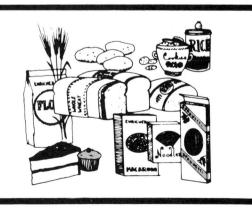

Figure 9.1. Four basic food groups.

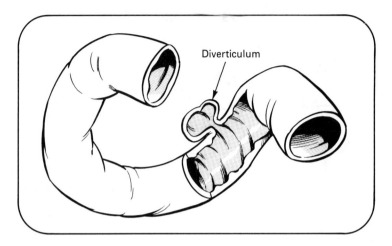

Figure 9.2(a). Diverticulosis.

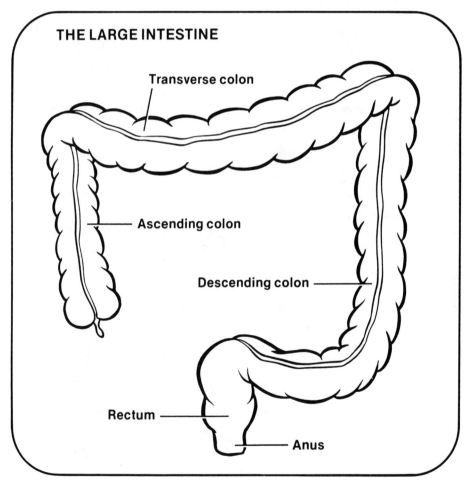

Figure 9.2(b). Normal large colon.

to 3000 cc of fluid to maintain the flow of urine and prevent stagnate bacteria from causing a bladder infection.

Fluid balance is a term which means that the amount of fluid taken in equals the amount of fluid lost from the body (Figure 9.3). The elderly person can reach a critical state and confusion can occur when problems develop that upset the fluid balance. Problems include those of diarrhea, vomiting, excessive perspiration, or excessive wound drainage. Fluids lost in these ways must be replaced as soon as possible in order to restore a fluid balance and important chemical elements such as chloride and potassium. The older person will also lose fluid with increased respiration due to respiratory disease, and by increased urination if taking diuretic medications. Confusion can result from any of these conditions where there is a depletion of body fluids which are not replaced.

Adequate Dietary Fiber

Many diets are deficient in fiber. This has become a national problem with the increased amount of processed food in our markets and grocery stores today. However, for the elderly person, the addition of fiber in the diet is a necessity due to the decreased bowel motility and the frequency of constipation.

Fiber adds roughage to the diet and increases bulk, which in turn improves the movement of waste products through the bowels. Because of this increase in bowel motility, fiber can also be an aid in preventing a diverticulum from developing and in preventing hemorrhoids. Both conditions develop when constipation is a problem.

Fiber in bran and fruits and vegetables is a help in preventing constipation in elderly people in nursing homes. Bran can be sprinkled over foods or eaten

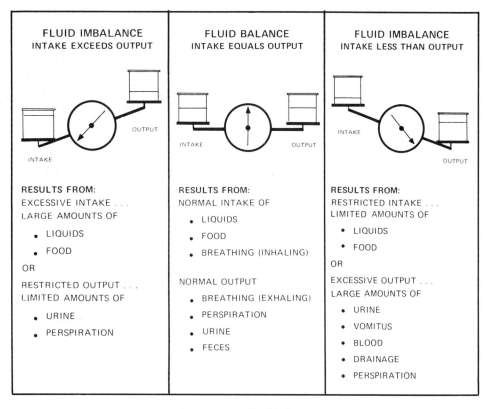

Figure 9.3. Fluid balance.

separately in the form of bran bread. Fresh vegetables and fruits also add bulk to the diet. An increase of these foods with an increase in water will help the elderly person prevent constipation.

Special or Modified Diets

Obesity is a common problem in older people who do not decrease caloric content when activity decreases. Low-caloric diets are needed to help the individual reduce body fat. Obesity is a risk factor for heart disease, high blood pressure, and osteoarthritis of the hip joints and knees. Increased caloric intake may also precipitate a late onset of diabetes. Obesity can be controlled with a low-caloric diet that is sufficient in all basic nutrients.

The person who is diabetic requires a balanced prescribed diet. Concentrated carbohydrates are restricted. The diet is balanced in the amounts of carbohydrates, fats, and proteins needed. The diabetic diet is a major part of the diabetic's treatment; therefore, foods that are not eaten must be reported in order to supplement these uneaten nutrients.

The low-sodium diet is prescribed for the person who must restrict the amount of salt intake. Usually, the diet is restricted to 200 to 500 mg of sodium. Restrictions of food include all table salt, milk, salted nuts, bacon, ham, and other products of high sodium content.

Other special diets may be prescribed for the elderly person, depending on the condition. The clear liquid diet is usually ordered for the person who has a gastrointestinal problem requiring rest to the stomach and intestines. The clear liquid diet contains those liquids that are clear: tea, broth, Jello, ginger ale, Seven-Up (usually, these must sit to eliminate bubbles). This diet is low on nutrients and is not continued beyond 2 to 3 days.

The full liquid diet allows those liquids that contain more substance and stay in the gastrointestinal tract longer: ice cream, strained soups, eggnog, juices, and milk . All diets are planned to provide some essential nutrients for the given condition. A resumption of a normal diet as soon as possible is preferred.

Pureed foods may be needed by elderly residents who have no teeth. If at all possible, it is better to try to have the person fitted with false dentures so that he or she can resume eating normal diets. However, some residents may never be able to regain a normal eating pattern. It is therefore important to encourage the person to eat foods served to maintain body nutrition and weight. Supplements may be necessary. These should be offered between meals and at bedtime.

Types of diets are summarized in Figure 9.4.

Other Factors to Consider at Mealtime

Mealtime should be a happy, pleasant time for residents. The geriatric nursing assistant should give full attention to the needs of each elderly person. If several nursing assistants are helping residents to eat in a congregated dining area, they should be involved in encouraging the residents to communicate with each other rather than using this time to communicate with another geriatric nursing assistant about the activities of their own personal lives. Other suggestions for mealtime are listed below.

TYPES OF DIETS GIVEN TO PATIENTS; WHAT THEY ARE AND WHY THEY ARE USED

Type of Diet	Description	Common Purpose
Regular	Provides all essentials of good nourishment in normal forms	For patients who do not need special diets
Clear liquid (hospital surgical)	Broth, tea, ginger ale, gelatin	Usually for patients who have had surgery or are very ill
Full liquid	Broth, tea, coffee, ginger ale, gelatin, strained fruit juices, liquids, custard, junket, ice cream, sherbet, pudding, soft-cooked eggs	For those unable to chew or swallow solid food
Light or soft	Foods soft in consistency; no rich or strongly flavored foods that could cause distress	Final stage for postoperative patient before resuming regular diet
Soft (mechanical)	Same foods as on a normal diet but chopped or strained	For patients who have difficulty in chewing or swallowing
Bland	Foods mild in flavor and easy to digest; omits spicy foods	Avoids irritation of the digestive tract, as with ulcer and colitis patients
Low residue	Foods low in fiber and bulk; omits foods difficult to digest	Spares the lower digestive tract, as with patients having rectal diseases
High calorie	Foods high in protein, carbohydrates, minerals, and vitamins	For underweight or malnourished patients
Low calorie	Low in cream, butter, cereals, desserts, and fats	For patients who need to lose weight
Diabetic	Precise balance of carbohydrates, protein, and fats, devised according to the needs of the individual patients	For diabetic patients; matches food intake with the insulin nutritional requirements
High protein	Meals supplemented with high-protein foods, such as meat, fish, cheese, milk, and eggs	Assists in the growth and repair of tissues wasted by disease
Low fat	Limited amounts of butter, cream, fats, and eggs	For patients who have difficulty digesting fats, as in gallbladder, cardiovascular, and liver disturbances
Low cholesterol	Low in eggs, whole milk, and meats	Helps regulate the amount of cholesterol in the blood
Low sodium (low salt)	Limited amounts of foods containing sodium; no salt allowed on tray	For patients whose circulation would be impaired by fluid retention; patients with certain heart or kidney conditions
Salt-free (sodium-free)	Completely without salt	
Tube feeding	Specialized formulas or liquid forms of nutrients given to the patient through a tube; follow with a glass of water at room temperature	For patients who, because of a condition such as oral surgery or decreased level of consciousness, cannot eat normally

Figure 9.4. Diets.

Nursing responses at mealtime that help the resident to maintain nutritional and fluid balance

The environment:

1. Remove clutter and unsightly, unnecessary items.
2. Provide a pleasant, cheerful environment.
3. Be sure that the area is clean.

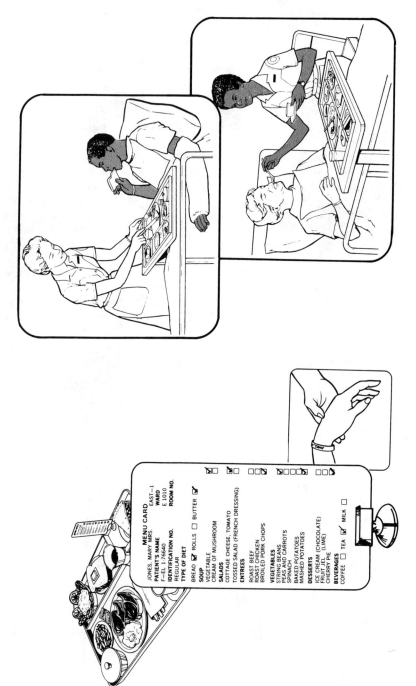

Figure 9.5.

The resident (Figure 9.5):

1. Assist the resident to prepare physically and psychologically: Allow enough time for oral hygiene, toileting, washing face and hands, and any other changes needed.
2. Be sure that resident has the right tray.
3. Assist with positioning and comfort; be sure that resident is free of any pain.
4. Assist with opening cartons, cutting meat, spreading butter on bread, and any actions difficult for the resident.
5. If assisting resident with eating, do not rush. Inform resident of foods on the tray; serve small amounts, alternating solids and liquids, from the tip of the spoon. Encourage resident to assist as much as possible. Use adaptive devices such as plate guards, enlarged utensil handles and adjustable utensils, cups with sipping seals, straws, and other devices as available.
6. Encourage the resident to eat what is served; be conscious of liquid intake; encourage liquids if unrestricted.
7. Learn resident's likes and dislikes regarding food.
8. Encourage family members to bring in favorite food if permitted by the facility.

THE CHOKING RESIDENT

Residents who have difficulty chewing and swallowing require particular attention. The geriatric nursing assistant should consult with the nurse in charge to set up a feeding plan for each of these residents and be skilled in how to relieve a resident who chokes and cannot speak or cough (Figure 9.6). The procedures for what to do if the resident requires emergency treatment follow this section.

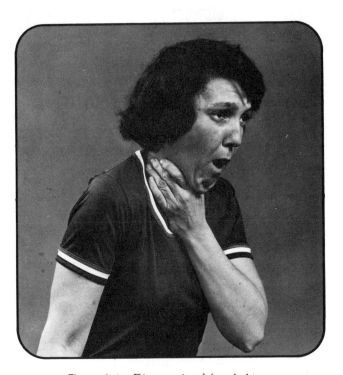

Figure 9.6. Distress signal for choking.

The geriatric nursing assistant should be skilled in the procedures for conscious and unconscious persons with an obstructed airway.

CHECKLIST FOR CHOKING PERSON WHO IS CONSCIOUS AND BECOMES UNCONSCIOUS

Note: During the practice of these skills, do not actually perform thrusts, finger sweeps, or rescue breathing on your partner. Rather, simulate these skills on your partner.

	Yes	*No*
1. *Assessment*		
a. Determine airway obstruction.		
—Ask, "Are you choking?"	—	—
—Determine if victim can speak, cough, or breathe.	—	—
b. *Situation:* Victim cannot speak, cough, or breathe. Call for help.		
—Shout "Help!"	—	—
2. *Heimlich maneuver.* Perform abdominal thrusts (Figure 9.7).		
a. Stand behind the victim.	—	—
b. Wrap arms around victim's waist.	—	—
c. Make a fist with one hand and place the thumb side against victim's abdomen in the midline slightly above the navel and well below the tip of the xiphoid.	—	—
d. Grasp fist with other hand.	—	—
e. Press into the victim's abdomen with quick upward thrusts.	—	—
f. Each thrust should be distinct and delivered with the intent of relieving the airway obstruction.	—	—
g. Repeat thrusts until object is expelled or the victim becomes unconscious.	—	—
h. No pressure should be exerted against the rib cage with the rescuer's forearms.	—	—

SELF-CHECK: CONSCIOUS CHOKING PERSON

Situation: Object cannot be removed and victim becomes unconscious. Please check appropriate response.

1. A person who coughs forcefully should be:
   ___ **a.** Given care for a completely blocked airway.
   ___ **b.** Left alone and watched.
2. A person who coughs weakly, has great difficulty breathing, and is turning blue should be:
   ___ **a.** Given care for a completely blocked airway.
   ___ **b.** Left alone and watched.
3. If a person is in distress, is not coughing, but can speak:
   ___ **a.** Try to remove an object from the airway.
   ___ **b.** Do not try to remove an object from the airway.

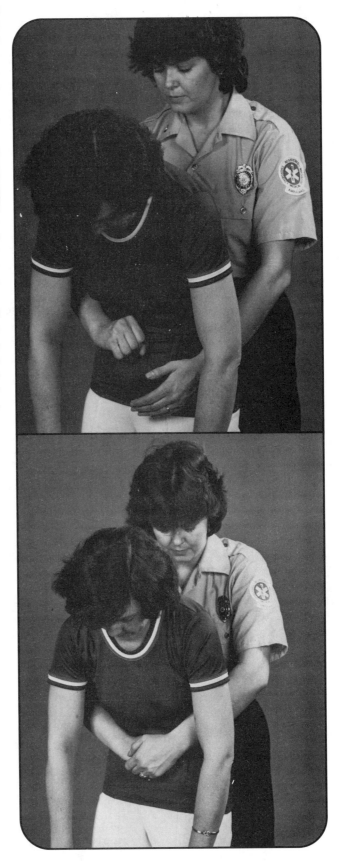

Figure 9.7. Heimlich manuever.

4. When you give abdominal thrusts, what part of your fist do you place against the victim?
   __ **a.** The palm side.
   __ **b.** The thumb side.

5. Where do you place your fist?
   __ **a.** Slightly above the navel but well below the tip of the xiphoid.
   __ **b.** Between the rib cage and the waist.

6. Abdominal thrusts are given quickly,
   __ **a.** Inward and upward.
   __ **b.** Straight back.

7. You are giving abdominal thrusts to a woman whose airway is completely blocked; then she begins to cough forcefully. You should:
   __ **a.** Continue to give abdominal thrusts.
   __ **b.** Stop right away.

8. If abdominal thrusts fail and the victim is still conscious, you should:
   __ **a.** Stop giving thrusts.
   __ **b.** Keep giving thrusts.

Check whether you will give thrusts to each victim of choking.

	Yes	*No*
9. Person coughing vigorously.	__	__
10. Person coughing weakly, making wheezing noises, and turning blue.	__	__
11. Person able to talk.	__	__
12. Person not able to talk.	__	__

13. You are giving abdominal thrusts to a choking victim who loses consciousness. You should:
   __ **a.** Continue to give abdominal thrusts.
   __ **b.** Sweep the mouth and attempt to ventilate.

Obstructed Airway: Unconscious Adult Victim

The first step for an unconscious person is the *airway* step—call for help; then tilt the head to open the airway. Next is the *breathing* step—check for breathing, and if the person is not breathing normally, try to give two full, slow breaths. If air *will* go into the lungs, continue with the *circulation* step—check the pulse. Give rescue breathing or CPR if needed.

If air will *not* go into the lungs when you try to give two full, slow breaths, retilt the head and try again—*you may not have tilted the head far enough*, and the tongue may be blocking the airway.

If the airway is partly blocked but you can force air into the lungs with long, slow breaths, do so. Do not try to remove an object if you can force air into the lungs. You may be able to keep the person alive until medical help arrives or the person recovers enough to begin coughing.

If the airway remains blocked after you have retilted the head and attempted to ventilate, perform *abdominal thrusts*. See figure 9.8(a) and 9.8(b). Straddle the victim's thighs, then put the heel of one hand on the victim's abdomen, in the midline slighty above the navel and well below the xiphoid, then put the other hand on top of the first. Point the fingers of the bottom hand toward the head. With your shoulders directly over the victim's abdomen, press inward and up-

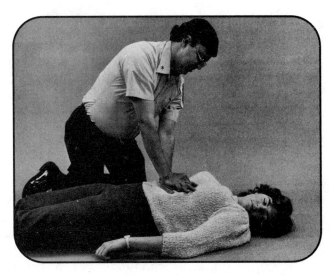

Figure 9.8(a).   Abdominal thrust technique used on a patient who is lying down.

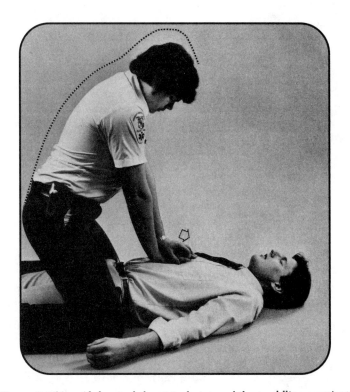

Figure 9.8(b).   Abdominal thrust technique while straddling a patient.

ward with 6 to 10 abdominal thrusts. Do not press to either side because you may injure the victim.

When you have completed the 6 to 10 abdominal thrusts, you should:

1. Move back to the victim's head and perform a finger sweep.
2. Attempt to ventilate, and if air still does not go in,
3. Perform another series of 6 to 10 abdominal thrusts.
4. Repeat the sequence until successful.

Remember, if you cannot inflate the lungs after retilting the head and trying again, an object is probably blocking the airway. Take these steps:

1. Perform abdominal thrusts (6 to 10).
2. Finger sweep.
3. Attempt to ventilate.
4. Repeat the sequence until it works.

Chest Thrusts: Unconscious Choking Victim

The chest thrust is an alternative to the abdominal thrust for unconscious victims as well as for conscious victims, but only for women in advanced stages of pregnancy or when the victim is too obese for the rescuer to apply abdominal thrusts effectively (Figures 9.9 and 9.10).

For giving chest thrusts to an unconscious person, the body position and hand position are the same as for chest compressions in CPR. See page 268 for a description of how to do it.

HEIMLICH MANEUVER: UNCONSCIOUS PERSON

	Yes	No
1. *Assessment*		
a. Position victim.		
—Turn victim on back as unit.	—	—
—Place victim face up with arms at side.	—	—
b. Call for help.		
—Shout '"Help!"' or if others respond, direct them to activate the EMS system.	—	—
2. *Foreign body check.* Perform finger sweep.		
a. Keep victim's face up.	—	—
b. Thumb in mouth, lift jaw and tongue (tongue-jaw lift). See Figure 9.11.	—	—
c. Sweep deeply into mouth with index finger from one cheek to the other. See Figure 9.12.	—	—
Situation: Object cannot be removed.		
3. *Breathing.* Attempt to ventilate.		
a. Open airway.	—	—
b. Seal mouth and nose.	—	—
c. Attempt to ventilate.	—	—
Situation: Airway is blocked.		
4. *Heimlich maneuver.* Perform abdominal thrusts.		
a. Straddle victim's thighs.	—	—
b. Place heel of one hand against victim's abdomen, in the midline slightly above navel and well below tip of xiphoid.	—	—
c. Place second hand directly over first hand.	—	—

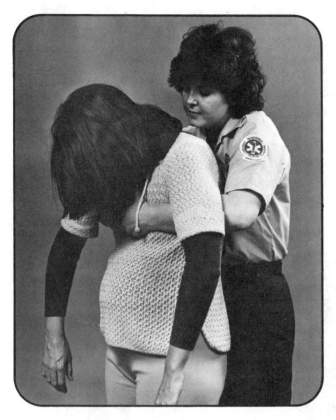

Figure 9.9. Chest thrust applied to a pregnant woman.

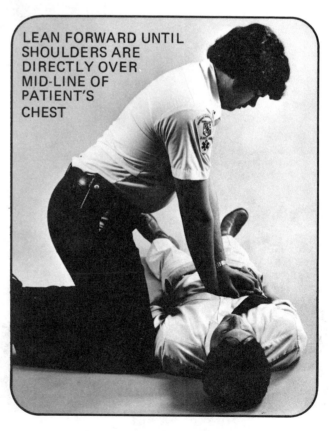

LEAN FORWARD UNTIL SHOULDERS ARE DIRECTLY OVER MID-LINE OF PATIENT'S CHEST

Figure 9.10. The chest thrust method can be used when the patient is lying on his back.

	Yes	No
d. Press into the abdomen with quick upward thrusts.	—	—
e. Perform 6 to 10 abdominal thrusts.	—	—
f. Each thrust should be distinct and delivered with the intent of relieving the foreign body obstruction.	—	—

5. *Foreign body check.* Perform finger sweep.

	Yes	No
a. Keep victim's face up.	—	—
b. Tongue-jaw lift to open mouth.	—	—
c. Sweep deeply into mouth with index finger from one cheek to the other.	—	—

Situation: Object still cannot be removed.

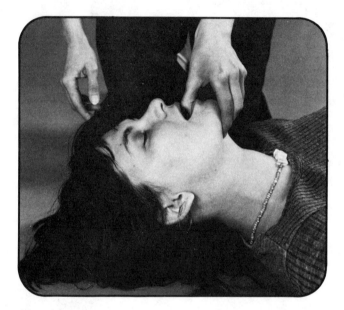

Figure 9.11.   Tongue-jaw lift.

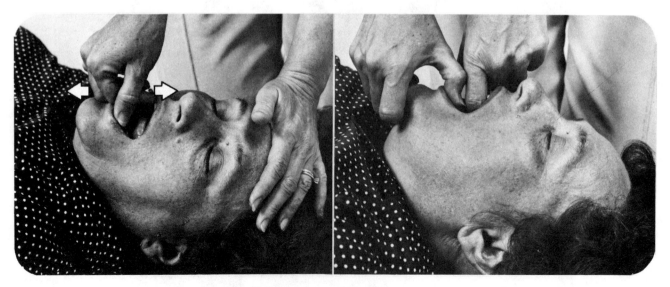

Figure 9.12.   Open the patient's mouth using the crossed–fingers technique. Use finger sweeps to remove foreign objects from the airway and the mouth.

	Yes	*No*
6. *Breathing.* Attempt ventilation.		
a. Open airway.	—	—
b. Seal mouth and nose.	—	—
c. Attempt to ventilate.	—	—
Situation: Airway is still blocked.		
7. *Sequencing.* Repeat sequence of steps 4 to 6 until successful.	—	—

The procedures for clearing the airway of an unconscious adult are summarized in Figure 9.13.

CHECKLIST FOR OBSTRUCTED AIRWAY: UNCONSCIOUS ADULT VICTIM

Situation: You have come upon a resident with a death-like appearance.

Note: During the practice of these skills, if a manikin is not used, do not actually perform thrusts, finger sweeps, or rescue breathing on your partner, but rather, simulate these skills. If a manikin is used for this practice session, simulate finger sweeps.

	Yes	*No*
1. *Assessment/airway*		
a. Determine unresponsiveness.		
—Tap or gently shake shoulder.	—	—
—Shout, "Are you okay?"	—	—
Situation: Victim is unresponsive.		
b. Call for help.		
—Shout "Help!"	—	—
c. Open the airway.		
—Use head-tilt/chin-lift maneuver.	—	—
2. *Breathing*		
a. Check breathing.		
—Maintain open airway.	—	—
—Look at chest; listen and feel for breathing (3 to 5 seconds).	—	—
Situation: Victim is not breathing.		
b. Attempt ventilation.		
—Maintain open airway.	—	—
—Seal mouth and nose properly.	—	—
—Attempt to ventilate.	—	—
Situation: Airway is blocked.		
c. Reattempt ventilation.		
—Retilt victim's head.	—	—
—Seal mouth and nose properly.	—	—
—Attempt to ventilate.	—	—
Situation: Airway is still blocked.		
d. Activate EMS system.		
—Direct someone to activate the EMS system!	—	—

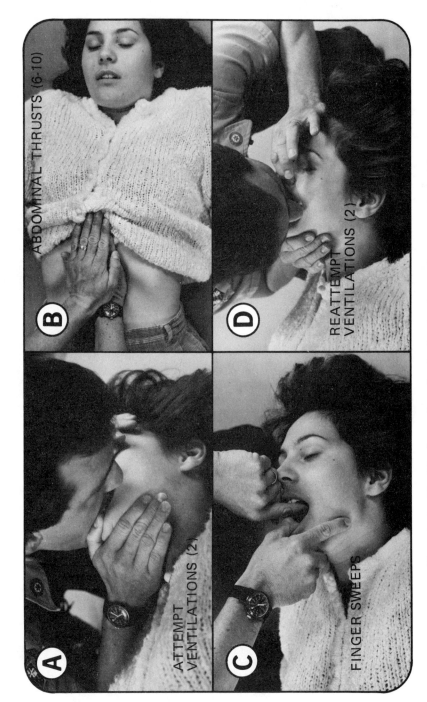

Figure 9.13. Combined procedures for clearing the airway of an unconscious adult.

198

	Yes	*No*

3. *Heimlich maneuver.* Perform abdominal thrusts.
   a. Straddle victim's thighs. — —
   b. Place heel of one hand against victim's abdomen, in the midline slightly above navel and well below tip of xiphoid. — —
   c. Place second hand directly over first hand. — —
   d. Press into the abdomen with quick, upward thrusts. — —
   e. Perform 6 to 10 abdominal thrusts. — —
   f. Each thrust should be distinct and delivered with the intent of relieving the foreign body obstruction. — —
4. *Foreign body check.* Perform finger sweep.
   a. Keep victim's face up. — —
   b. Tongue-jaw lift to open mouth. — —
   c. Sweep deeply into mouth with index finger from one cheek to the other. — —
   Situation: Object cannot be removed.
5. *Breathing.* Attempt ventilation.
   a. Open airway. — —
   b. Seal mouth and nose properly. — —
   c. Attempt to ventilate. — —
   Situation: Airway is still blocked.
6. *Sequencing.* Repeat sequence of steps 3 to 5 until successful. — —

SELF-CHECK: UNCONSCIOUS PERSON WITH OBSTRUCTED AIRWAY

Please check appropriate response.

1. The first step for an unconscious person is to:
   __ a. Look in the mouth for an object blocking the airway.
   __ b. Tilt the head and check for breathing.
2. If you cannot inflate the lungs the first time you try to give two full, slow breaths, you should:
   __ a. Retilt the head and try again.
   __ b. Give more breaths.
3. You try to give breaths and you can inflate the lungs, but it is difficult to do so. What can you do?
   __ a. Give breaths.
   __ b. Give abdominal thrusts.
4. To give abdominal thrusts, place the heel of the hand:
   __ a. Over the edge of the rib cage.
   __ b. Slightly above the navel and well below the tip of the xiphoid.
5. Placing your other hand on top of the first hand, give thrusts:
   __ a. Straight toward the ground.
   __ b. Inward and upward, toward the lungs.
6. You give 6 to 10 abdominal thrusts to an unconscious victim. After giving the thrusts, you should:
   __ a. Sweep with your finger.
   __ b. Attempt to ventilate.

7. When you use a finger sweep:
    ___ **a.** Tilt the head forward and press the tongue back with your thumb.
    ___ **b.** Grasp the tongue and lower jaw between your thumb and fingers, and lift.

8. Try to remove the object by:
    ___ **a.** Sweeping from side to side.
    ___ **b.** Poking straight into the throat.

9. After you sweep the mouth with a finger, the victim is still not breathing. Next you:
    ___ **a.** Try to give breaths.
    ___ **b.** Give 6 to 10 abdominal thrusts.

10. If you can inflate the lungs fully but think there may be an object in the airway:
    ___ **a.** Stop giving breaths and try to remove the object.
    ___ **b.** Keep giving breaths.

INTRAVENOUS FEEDINGS

Intravenous feedings are one way to provide fluids, nutrients, and medications to people who are too ill to take them by mouth (Figure 9.14). The intravenous route is also the most rapid way to get important elements into an acutely ill person. The procedure involved in administering intravenous solutions is done under sterile technique. Even though this procedure is done by licensed personnel, the nursing assistant can play a major role in observing the intravenous as she or he cares for the patient/resident. The nursing assistant should promptly report any unusual signs that the intravenous may be causing some undue stress to the resident either because of a local reaction at the site of the needle or by a general body reaction to the solutions being administered.

Review the checklist for the various kinds of problems that can occur with intravenous fluids. The term *infiltrate* should be one you know. Infiltration means the escape of the IV fluid from the vein into the surrounding tissue. Careful handling of the resident with an IV is necessary so that the needle does not become dislodged. An infiltrated IV requires that the IV be discontinued and must be restarted using another sterile IV set and another vein.

CHECKLIST FOR OBSERVING INTRAVENOUS FLUIDS

The nursing assistant checks for the following (Figure 9.15):

	Yes	*No*
1. Comfort of resident (as compared to time before IV)		
a. Free of pain at needle site	—	—
b. Free of swelling at needle site; needle anchored	—	—
c. Normal skin color at needle site (compared to site without IV)	—	—
d. Resident's respirations are unchanged (free of rapid breathing and chest pain)	—	—
e. Skin clear of rashes	—	—
f. Free of anxiety, restlessness	—	—

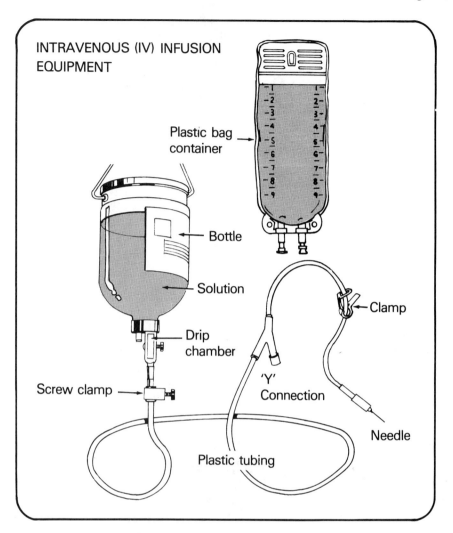

INTRAVENOUS (IV) INFUSION EQUIPMENT

Plastic bag container

Bottle

Solution

Drip chamber

Screw clamp

Clamp

'Y' Connection

Needle

Plastic tubing

Figure 9.14.

	Yes	No
2. Tubing		
a. Intact, no leaks	—	—
b. No kinks	—	—
c. Free of tangles	—	—
d. Not under resident	—	—
3. Drip chamber (check with supervisor)		
a. Filling correctly	—	—
b. Correct rate of drip	—	—

Licensed personnel are responsible for all of the above and the following:

4. Solution container		
a. Has name of correct solution	—	—
b. Correct number on container	—	—
c. Date and time on container as necessary	—	—
5. Proper recording of solutions on resident's I and O record	—	—

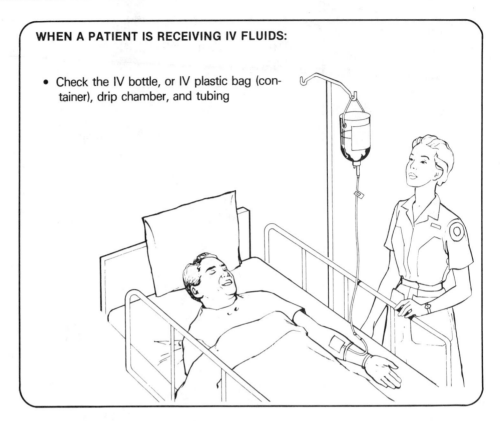

WHEN A PATIENT IS RECEIVING IV FLUIDS:

• Check the IV bottle, or IV plastic bag (container), drip chamber, and tubing

Figure 9.15.

RESIDENTS WITH TUBES: GENERAL NURSING CARE

Tubes are used to connect an interior part of the body with the exterior. There are many different types of tubes that have been inserted into patients. Some are for feeding purposes (Figure 9.16) and some are for drainage purposes (Figure 9.17). A nasogastric tube is one that is passed to a person's stomach through the nose, down the esophagus to the stomach. Its main purpose is to provide nourishment. Prepared formulas and other liquids are instilled into the tube at regular intervals. These feedings take the place of the diet that otherwise would be eaten normally.

General Guidelines for Nursing Care for Residents with Tubes

1. Know where the tube is and how far it extends into the body.
2. Tubes inserted during surgery require sterile techniques in their care.
3. Keep tubes in the open and not coiled under the resident.
4. Check the resident for comfort; report any changes in vital signs; be alert for fever; check for irritation at the site of the tube (redness, swelling).

The following discussion for nursing care of residents receiving tube feedings is included to provide information for the geriatric nursing assistant. There may be a time when the nursing assistant will assist the licensed nurse in doing the procedure.

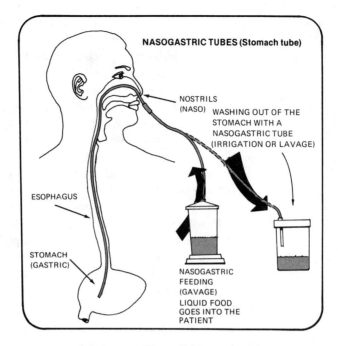

Figure 9.16.

Nursing Care of Residents with Nasogastric Tube Feedings

These tasks are performed by licensed personnel, but nursing assistants may assist.

1. Check physician's order for type of feeding, amount, and times.
2. Have resident in comfortable position, usually in the sitting position. Explain procedure.

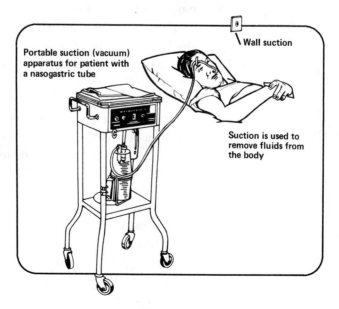

Figure 9.17.

3. Wash hands; assemble all equipment and the feeding (usually 300 to 500 ml at room temperature).

4. Feeding can be in a plastic container with drip chamber similar to an IV solution.

5. Licensed professional nurses must check to be sure that the tube is in the stomach. This is usually determined by undoing the clamp on the tube and withdrawing a small amount of stomach content via syringe. Tube must be well anchored over the nose with tape.

6. If not in a continuous drip container, feeding is instilled by a 20- to 50-cc syringe or via a funnel. Prior to instilling feeding, tube should be checked for patency with 15 to 30 ml of water. Water and feedings flow in by gravity or the flow is controlled by a pump.

7. Following feeding, tube should again be cleansed with the instillation of 15 to 30 ml of water. The tube is clamped.

8. Assure resident's comfort. Leave resident in a position that aids in the digestion process. Report any symptoms, such as fullness or nausea, choking, diarrhea, or constipation.

9. Record feeding on intake and output sheet.

10. Clean up equipment and put away.

11. Always provide for good mouth care for residents with nasogastric tubes to help prevent any infections of the mouth and to add to comfort.

CHECKLIST FOR NASOGASTRIC TUBE FEEDINGS

Note: Performed by licensed personnel only.

	Yes	No
1. Check doctor's orders for kind of feeding, amount, time.	—	—
2. Wash hands; gather equipment as applicable.		
a. Plastic bag of tube feeding at room temperature	—	—
b. Funnel, feeding container	—	—
c. Water for cleansing tubing at room temperature	—	—
d. Tube feeding pump, if ordered	—	—
3. Unclamp tube, instill 15 to 30 ml of water; pinch tube to prevent air from entering.	—	—
4. Check anchor of tube and condition of skin in nostrils.	—	—
5. Have professional check placement of tube in stomach.	—	—
6. Hook up funnel or plastic bag.	—	—
7. Set clamp on tubing to allow formula to run slowly or administer through funnel slowly or set pump according to order.	—	—
8. Observe resident for tolerance, nausea, fullness.	—	—
9. Report any unusual symptoms.	—	—
10. Help resident to feel at ease.	—	—
11. Provide for resident's comfort throughout procedure.	—	—
12. Instill 15 to 30 ml of water after feeding.	—	—
13. Place clamp on tube and attach tube to patient's clothing, free of tension.	—	—
14. Clean up equipment and bedside unit.	—	—

	Yes	No
15. Record feeding on intake and output.	—	—
16. Provide frequent mouth care.	—	—

Observations for the Nursing Assistant

	Yes	No
1. Privacy is maintained.	—	—
2. Elevated head position.	—	—
3. Frequent mouth care provided.	—	—
4. Comfort maintained.	—	—
5. Feeding is dripping slowly.	—	—
6. Observation is made for fullness, nausea, and tolerance.	—	—
7. Observations are made for variations in defecation: diarrhea, constipation.	—	—
8. Tubing is free of kinks.	—	—
9. Any unusual symptoms are reported immediately.	—	—

Gastrostomy Feedings

A gastrostomy feeding is the instillation of liquid nourishment through a tube that was surgically inserted into the resident's stomach. Gastrostomies are usually done because of some problem in the mouth or in the esophagus. Sometimes the gastrostomy is temporary, other times, in case of removal of the esophagus due to cancer, the gastrostomy is permanent. Psychological considerations must be made and care given to help the resident with any emotional problems that may result. For instance, initially it is very difficult for a person with a permanent gastrostomy to eat with others who can chew and eat normally.

Assessment of the skin around the gastrostomy tube is necessary to prevent any accumulation of drainage and skin breakdown. Any redness or broken skin should be reported immediately. Symptoms of fullness, nausea, diarrhea, or constipation should also be given immediate attention. Feedings are usually the same as nasogastric feedings, 300 to 500 cc.

Note: The geriatric nursing assistant may not be permitted to do gastrostomy feedings; the state law and the facility policy must be known. However, it is important for the nursing assistant to know how to care for the resident with a gastrostomy. You may be permitted to assist the licensed person in the procedure.

CHECKLIST FOR OBSERVATION OF A GASTROSTOMY FEEDING*

Note: Nursing assistant must know what he or she is permitted to do in this procedure.

Licensed Personnel

	Yes	No
1. Checked doctor's order for kind, amount, time of feeding.	—	—

*Check facility policy. The nursing assistant may not be permitted to do feedings but should understand how it is done and what to observe and report.

	Yes	No
2. Washed hands, gathered equipment as ordered.		
a. Plastic bag of tube feeding for slow drip at room temperature; pump if ordered.	—	—
b. Funnel, feeding container.	—	—
c. Water for cleansing tube at room temperature.	—	—
3. Provided privacy.	—	—
4. Explained procedure.	—	—
5. Checked anchor of tube.	—	—
6. Checked condition of skin around tube.	—	—
7. Unclamped tube, instilled 15 to 30 ml of water; pinched tube to prevent air from entering.	—	--
8. Set up equipment, either plastic bag for slow drip or funnel for slow instillation of fluid.	—	—
9. Observed resident for tolerance, nausea, fullness.	—	—
10. Reported any unusual symptoms.	—	—
11. Helped resident feel at ease.	—	—
12. Provided for resident's comfort throughout procedure.	—	—
13. Instilled 15 to 30 ml of water after feeding.	—	—
14. Placed clamp on tube and secured in place.	—	—
15. Cleaned up equipment and bedside unit.	—	—
16. Recorded feeding on intake and output.	—	—
17. Provided frequent mouth care.	—	—

Observations by the Geriatric Nursing Assistant

	Yes	No
1. Privacy maintained.	—	—
2. Tube is anchored.	—	—
3. Skin around the tube is free of irritation.	—	—
4. Feeding is dripping slowly.	—	—
5. Tubing is free and has no kinks.	—	—
6. Resident is observed for tolerance, nausea, and fullness.	—	—
7. Frequent mouth care is provided.	—	—
8. Resident's comfort is maintained.	—	—
9. Any unusual symptoms are reported.	—	—

KEY POINTS

1. Nutrition and fluid balances are important to the state of wellness and resistance to infections/disease.
2. Elderly residents can easily go into a fluid imbalance.
3. Careful monitoring of intake and output of all residents is necessary, especially those losing fluid by diarrhea, vomiting, or related disorders.
4. Develop empathy and provide emotional support for residents who cannot eat normally. Provide careful feeding procedures to those who have trouble swallowing.
5. Know your facility's policy on what procedures you can assist with when residents receive feedings by tube.

6. Know the signs and symptoms to watch for when residents are receiving IV feedings and tube feedings. Report these immediately.
7. Practice your emergency procedures for relieving any person of airway obstruction.

SELF-CHECK

1. Define fluid balance. What conditions can easily cause an imbalance in an elderly person?

2. Mrs. Brown just returned from the hospital where she was treated for pneumonia. She is eating about half of her diet and does not want to drink her liquids. Why should you report this immediately?

3. The doctor begins intravenous feedings on Mrs. Brown (see question 2). What are four signs you will watch for while the IV is running?

4. Mrs. Brown becomes progressively weaker. The IVs are stopped and her family wants her to receive nasogastric feedings. What nursing assistant responses will you provide if a tube feeding is started?

SUGGESTED ACTIVITIES

1. Know your facility policies for weighing residents. Weigh carefully and be sure to report those residents who are losing weight. A plan should be developed for helping residents gain weight.
2. Invite a nutritionist from a nursing home to discuss common problems and solutions of nutritional deficits elderly people experience.
3. Investigate what is done in your facility to help increase fiber in residents' diets. What kind of treatment is given for constipation? Does it work?
4. Invite a throat specialist to discuss the best way to help a person with a swallowing problem to eat. What kind of exercises might be helpful?
5. Investigate the kind of devices your facility has to help a person with feeding. Visit a rehabilitation unit that helps to rehabilitate individuals who are handicapped and require devices to help them eat.

CLINICAL APPLICATION

1. Using the problem-solving worksheet provided, select a resident for whom you provide care who has a nutritional/fluid balance problem. Review the resident's chart and talk with the nurse in charge in order to complete the worksheet. Share the situation with your class and your instructor.

2. After you have mastered the steps for performing chest thrusts on an unconscious person, practice what you would do for a victim who is in one of the following situations, using the checklist provided.
   a. The conscious victim begins to cough after abdominal thrusts.
   b. The conscious victim is sitting in a chair when he or she begins choking.
   c. The rescuer removes the object from the unconscious victim while performing finger sweeps.
   d. The unconscious victim begins to cough.
   e. The rescuer can successfully ventilate the unconscious victim.

3. After you have mastered the steps for clearing an obstructed airway in an unconscious adult victim, practice what you would do for a victim who is in one of the following situations, using the checklist provided. (Have your partner tell you what you find as you progress through the steps.)
   a. Rescuer can inflate the victim's lungs.
   b. Object is removed during the finger sweep.

WORKSHEET

Nursing Responses to a Problem in Nutritional and/or Fluid Balance

Resident's Diagnosis	Nutritional/ Fluid Problem	Fluid Intake for 24 Hours	Fluid Output for 24 Hours	Food Eaten in 24 Hours

Nursing responses: What actions were taken to resolve the problem?

Evaluation: What nursing responses worked? Include how to prevent the problem from re-occurring.

WORKSHEET

Obstructed Airway: Unconscious Person

	Yes	No
1. *Assessment*		
a. Position victim.		
—Turn victim on back as unit.	—	—
—Place victim face up with arms at side.	—	—
b. Call for help.		
—Shout "Help!" or if others respond, direct them to activate the EMS System.	—	—
2. *Foreign body check.* Perform finger sweep.		
a. Keep victim's face up.	—	—
b. Thumb in mouth, lift jaw and tongue (tongue-jaw lift).	—	—
c. Sweep deeply into mouth with index finger from one cheek to the other.	—	—
Situation: Object cannot be removed.		
3. *Breathing.* Attempt to ventilate.		
a. Open airway.	—	—
b. Seal mouth and nose.	—	—
c. Attempt to ventilate.	—	—
Situation: Airway is blocked.		
4. *Heimlich Maneuver.* Perform abdominal thrusts.		
a. Straddle victim's thighs.	—	—
b. Place heel of one hand against victim's abdomen, in the midline slightly above navel and well below tip of xiphoid.	—	—
c. Place second hand directly over first hand.	—	—
d. Press into the abdomen with quick upward thrusts.	—	—
e. Perform 6 to 10 abdominal thrusts.	—	—
f. Each thrust should be distinct and delivered with the intent of relieving the foreign body obstruction.	—	—
5. *Foreign body check.* Perform finger sweep.		
a. Keep victim's face up.	—	—
b. Tongue-jaw lift to open mouth.	—	—
c. Sweep deeply into mouth with index finger from one cheek to the other.	—	—
Situation: Object still cannot be removed.		
6. *Breathing.* Attempt ventilation.		
a. Open airway.	—	—
b. Seal mouth and nose.	—	—
c. Attempt to ventilate.	—	—
Situation: Airway is still blocked.		
7. *Sequencing.* Repeat sequence of steps 4 to 6 until successful.	—	—

SELF-CHECK WORKSHEET

	Yes	No

1. *Assessment/airway*
   - a. Determine unresponsiveness.
     - —Tap or gently shake shoulder.   —   —
     - —Shout, "Are you okay?"   —   —
   - *Situation:* Victim is unresponsive.
   - b. Call for help.
     - —Shout, "Help!"   —   —
   - c. Open the airway.
     - —Use head-tilt/chin-lift maneuver.   —   —
2. *Breathing*
   - a. Check breathing.
     - —Maintain open airway.   —   —
     - —Look at chest; listen and feel for breathing (3 to 5 seconds).   —   —
   - *Situation:* Victim is not breathing.
   - b. Attempt ventilation.
     - —Maintain open airway.   —   —
     - —Seal mouth and nose properly.   —   —
     - —Attempt to ventilate.   —   —
   - *Situation:* Airway is blocked.
   - c. Reattempt ventilation.
     - —Retilt victim's head.   —   —
     - —Seal mouth and nose properly.   —   —
     - —Attempt to ventilate.   —   —
   - *Situation:* Airway is still blocked.
   - d. Activate EMS system.
     - —Direct someone to activate the EMS system!   —   —
3. *Heimlich maneuver.* Perform abdominal thrusts.
   - a. Straddle victim's thighs.   —   —
   - b. Place heel of one hand against victim's abdomen, in the midline slightly above navel and well below tip of xiphoid.   —   —
   - c. Place second hand directly over first hand.   —   —
   - d. Press into the abdomen with quick, upward thrusts.   —   —
   - e. Perform 6 to 10 abdominal thrusts.   —   —
   - f. Each thrust should be distinct and delivered with the intent of relieving the foreign body obstruction.   —   —
4. *Foreign body check.* Perform finger sweep.
   - a. Keep victim's face up.   —   —
   - b. Tongue-jaw lift to open mouth.   —   —
   - c. Sweep deeply into mouth with index finger from one cheek to the other.   —   —
   - *Situation:* Object cannot be removed.
5. *Breathing.* Attempt ventilation.
   - a. Open airway.   —   —
   - b. Seal mouth and nose properly.   —   —
   - c. Attempt to ventilate.   —   —
   - *Situation:* Airway is still blocked.
6. *Sequencing.* Repeat sequence of steps 3 to 5 until successful.   —   —

10 BLADDER AND BOWEL MANAGEMENT

TERMINAL PERFORMANCE OBJECTIVE

Given geriatric nursing assistant measures for bladder and bowel management, be able to apply these measures to clients with bladder and bowel problems.

Enabling Objectives

1. Define urinary incontinence.
2. Identify five factors that contribute to urinary incontinence in the elderly person.
3. List eight nursing measures that may help an elderly person to control urinary incontinence.
4. Define constipation.
5. Identify five factors that may contribute to constipation.
6. List five nursing measures that may help an elderly person to control a tendency for constipation.
7. Apply nursing measures to help clients regain bladder and bowel control.

REVIEW SECTION

The topics the geriatric nursing assistant should review with the instructor are the age-related changes of the urinary and digestive systems and the bodily requirements for fluid balance and good nutrition.

MEETING CHANGES IN THE URINARY SYSTEM THAT AFFECT BLADDER FUNCTIONING IN THE ELDERLY

Urinary incontinence is a common problem for elderly people. It usually affects women more than men. Urinary incontinence is a loss of control over urination, resulting in an involuntary release of urine. Incontinence affects people living in the community as well as people in institutions. It has been estimated that 40 to 60 percent of the residents of nursing homes are affected.

Factors that contribute to this problem are the following (Figure 10.1): poor neurological sensation or impulses to the bladder; bladder muscle weakness; obstruction blocking the flow of urine; urinary tract infections; mental confusion; medications that increase urinary flow, such as diuretics; fecal impaction; and environmental obstruction, such as difficulty in getting to toileting facilities. Poor vision and limited mobility also contribute to a person's difficulty in getting to the bathroom in time.

The elderly person has a decreased time lapse between the sensation to void and the need to void. This means that there is very little time to get to the bathroom after a person realizes that the bladder needs to be emptied. This lack of time is a distinct difference from the sensations felt by younger people and a difference the care giver should always remember. The older person does not deliberately become incontinent. This experience is very embarrassing and can cause the older person to become upset, especially if the care giver is not considerate and may blame the older person for not saying something sooner.

The person with incontinence who is mentally aware will welcome the geriatric nursing assistant who wants to help work out a plan to control the incontinence. It is very important that the elderly person wants to correct the problem and will try to do what is necessary. It is almost impossible to help a client overcome incontinence if he or she does not or cannot cooperate.

The geriatric nursing assistant must examine his or her own attitude about helping a client who is incontinent. An optimistic attitude is essential. The optimism must then be conveyed to the client. It is equally essential that *all* staff members concerned with care of the client participate in the plan of bladder retraining and have the same optimistic attitude. Positive reinforcement shared with the client will provide the encouragement needed to regain urinary control.

The client who is to be helped with urinary control requires a thorough physical assessment to rule out underlying problems. The physician in charge will need to learn if there is a neurological problem or if there is an infection that may

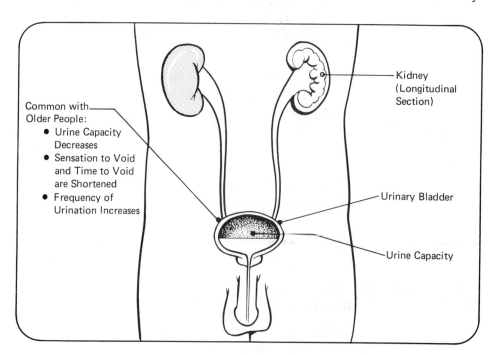

Figure 10.1. Urinary system.

be causing the incontinence. Once the assessment is completed and a clearance is given to help the client regain urinary control, the entire nursing staff needs to follow the facility's procedure for bladder retraining. A worksheet has been provided which the geriatric nursing assistant can help to complete on clients who will be participating in bladder retraining.

Geriatric Nursing Assistant Responses

1. Before starting bladder retraining, the client's voiding history should be noted for 48 to 72 hours to learn how often and how much is voided. A record should be kept on the times and amounts.

2. An intake record should be started to record how much fluid is taken within the same time periods. A comparison can be made between the amount of fluid intake compared to the amount of output. Note how much later the client voids after drinking fluids.

3. Offer fluids at least every 2 hours to help the client compensate for the decreased thirst sensation. A decreased thirst sensation is common to aging people.

4. Monitor urinary output. The bladder should be expanded to hold 250 ml (or cc).

5. A record can then be started to provide fluids and help the client to void. This means getting the client to the bathroom or on the bedpan as needed before the expected time of voiding. The time should gradually be increased to help the bladder expand and to regain normal functioning.

6. Provide (or offer) protective padding for use during the process of retraining. Some clients may want to wear some protection all the time to prevent leakage and avoid any embarrassment.

7. Provide an environment free of clutter so that there is easy access to the bathroom if client ambulates.

8. Assist the client to the bathroom at least every 2 hours and gradually increase time intervals as tolerated.

9. Give praise to clients who show some improvement.

10. Maintain an optimistic attitude. Communicate progress to all staff members and encourage their participation to assist the client in bladder management.

MEETING CHANGES IN THE DIGESTIVE SYSTEM THAT AFFECT BOWEL FUNCTIONING IN THE ELDERLY

Problems related to the large bowel (Figure 10.2) are common among the elderly. A review of the digestive system and age-related changes indicate that the older person's bowel has less motility. Peristalsis, the wavelike contraction of the bowel that moves the fecal contents along for elimination, is decreased.

Constipation

Constipation is a condition of decreased fecal elimination; the person's bowel movements are less than usual. Common causes of constipation are: poor nutrition and liquid intake, depression and other mental conditions, lesions of the bowel, and side effects of drugs. If constipation is not helped, a fecal impaction can occur. Any suspicion of constipation should be reported immediately.

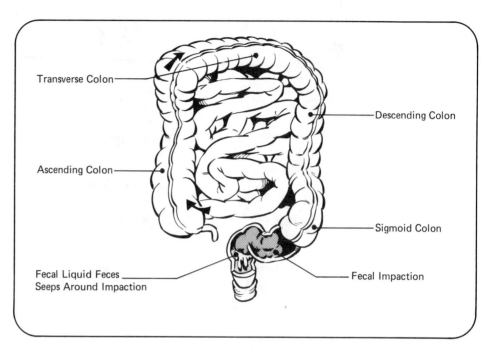

Figure 10.2. Bowel functioning.

Fecal Incontinence

The most common reason for fecal incontinence is fecal impaction. Liquid feces seep around the hard, dry, packed feces. Fecal incontinence may also occur from diarrhea, which is elimination of liquid feces usually caused by infection or drug intake. Diarrhea should be reported immediately.

Geriatric Nursing Assistant Responses

The geriatric nursing assistant can assist with preventing constipation in elderly clients. If the elderly person has repeated episodes of constipation or fecal impaction, a history should be obtained to determine what helps the person have normal bowel movements. The worksheet provided for history taking has the kind of questions that will be helpful in planning to assist the elderly person to overcome constipation. Other geriatric nursing assistant responses are:

1. Encourage the intake of 2000 to 2500 cc of fluids daily, including water, prune juice, and other fruit juices.
2. Add bulk, possibly bran, to diet (needs the doctor's order).
3. Increase physical exercise and mobility as much as possible.
4. Ask the charge nurse about a stool softener which can be ordered for the client.
5. Ask the charge nurse if medications may be contributing to the constipation.
6. Monitor bowel movements and report anything unusual, such as bleeding, immediately.

KEY POINTS

1. The positive attitude of the geriatric nursing assistant can contribute to assisting clients with bladder and bowel management.
2. Urinary incontinence is not a part of aging, although changes due to aging may contribute to the incontinence.
3. Both urinary and bowel problems are common among the elderly.
4. There are nursing assistant responses that can assist elderly clients to manage urinary and bowel problems.
5. All nursing staff members must work together to make the management care plans of clients effective.

SELF-CHECK

1. Mrs. Jones was never incontinent of urine or feces until last week. Now she says she cannot get to the bathroom before voiding a small amount. She hasn't had a satisfactory bowel movement for 5 days. What could be causing the urinary incontinence?

2. Mr. Whitehead has very bad vision. He walks with a cane because of his weak left side. He prides himself because he asks for very little assistance. Suddenly he has had trouble in getting to the bathroom before voiding. Suggest nursing measures to help him with his incontinence.

3. A thin elderly client always complains of constipation. After checking on her eating and drinking habits, you found that she only had 1200 cc of fluid and ate only soft foods. Suggest nursing measures to help overcome her constipation.

SUGGESTED ACTIVITIES

1. Talk with your charge nurse about clients who have been helped with incontinence and constipation. Note what kinds of nursing assisting measures were helpful.
2. Review the nursing assisting responses for residents with indwelling catheters. Make a list of actions the geriatric nursing assistant can do to help prevent complications.
3. Check on your facility's policies for bladder retraining after a person has had a catheter removed. Compare them to the suggestions in this unit.

4. Discuss what kinds of signs and symptoms should be immediately reported which indicate a problem with the elimination of urine and feces.

CLINICAL APPLICATION

Select a resident with urinary incontinence and a resident with constipation. Using the worksheets provided to obtain information about the residents, apply the geriatric nursing assistant measures to assist them.

WORKSHEET

History of Client's Voiding Pattern

Resident: _____   Diagnosis: _____
        (first name only)

Description of the problem:

1. Length of incontinence: Days ____ Months ____ Years ____
2. What is/are probable cause(s)?

3. Client knows when he/she has to void. Yes ____ No ____
4. Client can use: Bathroom   Yes ____   No ____
                 Commode   Yes ____   No ____
                 Bedpan   Yes ____   No ____
5. Client has additional conditions: (Check those that apply.)
    Poor vision ____   Walks with limited mobility ____
    Requires walker ____   Requires wheelchair ____
6. Intake for 48 to 72 hours: (Record amounts [in cc or ml] and kind.)

	Date/Time	Date/Time	Date/Time
Breakfast			
Lunch			
Dinner			
Between meals			
Nighttime			

7. Output for 48 to 72 hours. Record amount under each date and enter time and amount. After recording the output, indicate "C" for controlled voiding in bathroom, commode, bedpan; indicate "I" for incontinent. See the example below.

	Date/Time	Date/Time	Date/Time
AM (7–3)			
PM (3–11)			
Night (11–7)			

Example:

	Date/Time
AM (7–3)	200 cc C 7:30 A q.s. I 12 N 100 cc C 2 P
PM (3–11)	
Night (11–7)	

8. Look at intake amounts for 48 to 72 hours. Has client taken in at least 2000 ml? Does he or she need more liquids?

9. Make a list of liquids client likes:

10. State what will be done to help client.

11. Talk with charge nurse about updating the nursing care plan with nursing measures to be taken to prevent incontinence.

WORKSHEET

Bowel Management

Resident: _____   Diagnosis: _____
     (first name only)

Description of the problem:

1. Length of time of constipation: Days __ Months __ Years __
2. What is/are probable cause(s)?

3. When does client usually have B.M.?   ____   ____
                                              AM   PM

    After meals?   Yes __   No __

4. What has helped in the past?

      Prune juice ___   Fruits ___   Other _____

5. What is the consistency of the bowel movement?

6. Fluid intake for 48 hours: (Keep record of cc or ml.)

	Date/Time	Date/Time
AM (7–3)		
PM (3–11)		
Night (11–7)		
	Total ____	Total ____

7. Does client need more fluids? Yes __ No __
   (intake should be at least 2000 cc daily)
8. What kind of fluids does client like:

   Juices _____   Other fluids _____

9. Will bran be added to meals? Yes __ No __
   (Will need doctor's order.)

10. Will exercise be increased? Yes __ No __

11. Talk with charge nurse about updating the nursing care plan with nursing measures to be taken to prevent constipation.

11

COMMON DISEASES
AND DISABILITIES
OF THE ELDERLY

In this unit the geriatric nursing assistant will learn responses that are specific to people with certain diseases and disabilities. The diseases and disabilities discussed in this unit are common among elderly residents of nursing homes. The geriatric nursing assistant should approach each resident with the philosophy of care discussed in the first unit, regardless of the disease or disability and remember that each person lives with his or her chronic condition in a unique way. The underlying goal of giving care is to help people to function as independently as possible despite any disease or disability. One of the most challenging situations the geriatric nursing assistant will encounter is caring for the cognitively impaired client discussed in the first part of this unit.

Alzheimer's Disease and Related Disorders: Age-Related Changes

TERMINAL PERFORMANCE OBJECTIVE

Given information, guidelines, and specific nursing responses for cognitively impaired people, be able to assist family members and provide nursing responses to residents who have cognitive impairment.

Enabling Objectives

1. Define cognitive impairment.
2. Explain the impact that Alzheimer's disease has on the client and the client's family.
3. Differentiate between reversible and irreversible dementia. Provide examples of each.
4. Define "sundowning syndrome," hallucination, wandering behavior, delirium, agitation, and catastrophic reactions.
5. Outline geriatric nursing assistant responses to respond to people with: sundowning syndrome, hallucinations, wandering behavior, delirium, and agitation.

6. Identify two conditions that are related to Alzheimer's disease because of symptoms that eventually occur.
7. Practice communications to be used with a cognitively impaired person.
8. Develop a list of geriatric nursing assistant responses in caring for clients with Alzheimer's and related disorders (including confusion and depression).
9. Select a cognitively impaired person and provide geriatric nursing assistant responses.

REVIEW SECTION

The topics the geriatric nursing assistant should review with the instructor are the nervous system and age-related changes.

ALZHEIMER'S DISEASE

Alzheimer's disease (AD) was identified in 1906 by a German neurologist, Alois Alzheimer. The disease is characterized by a progressive degeneration of the brain, which results in memory loss and confusion. It has been estimated that 5 to 7 percent of the population over 65 years of age will be affected with a dementia of the Alzheimer type (SDAT). A dementia is a condition of deteriorating mentality. Researchers in the fields of neurology and psychiatry have grouped dementias into two categories, primary and secondary. A primary dementia is one with no known cause, is untreatable, and is irreversible. Alzheimer's is a primary dementia. The secondary type of dementia is one that is treatable and reversible if diagnosed early enough. Examples of secondary dementias are hypothyroidism and alcoholic psychosis.

The essential feature of Alzheimer's disease (AD) is the loss of intellectual abilities severe enough to interfere with social and occupational functioning. This deteriorating ability of intellectual functions is also known as cognitive impairment. Cognitive refers to cognition, the quality of knowing. It has been estimated that 50 percent of the clients in institutions of care have Alzheimer-type symptoms. As the older population increases, this percentage is expected to rise accordingly.

Alzheimer's disease is not part of aging. Older people do have some forgetfulness, but most people forget from time to time. The symptoms that distinguish the onset of Alzheimer's disease occur between 50 and 69 years of age. Clients have a fairly rapid decline with death occurring usually 5 to 10 years after symptoms occur, although people have lived longer.

The onset of symptoms may be fairly slow and not noticeable at first, but over a 5- to 10-year period, a young, vigorous midlife adult can become a person unknown to himself or herself and to significant people who care. Clients with Alzheimer's disease live shorter lives than would be projected for them otherwise. The last years cause sadness, guilt, anger, and confusion for both the care givers and the clients.

Theories about Causes

There are a number of theories now under research about causes of Alzheimer's disease. These center on the role of heredity, autoimmune reactions to toxin produced by one's own body, slow-acting viruses, and neurotransmitter deficits (decreased amounts of choline acetyltransferase needed to transmit across neurons). A great deal of research is going on throughout the country on Alzheimer's disease. Scientists feel that help will come in the near future just as it has for many other devastating diseases.

Five major areas of change are usually seen in Alzheimer clients. These are listed as follows:

Area of memory (early): short-term memory becomes disrupted; some hesitancy with speech and writing; poor ability to concentrate

Area of memory (later): cannot retain memory, becomes very forgetful; tries to cover up forgetfulness; mood changes occur because of forgetfulness

Area of spatial disorientation: difficulty interpreting spatial concepts, such as reading maps, parking a car; appears uncoordinated in the use of space; has difficulty using tools (i.e., scissors); may become socially isolated and depressed

Area of personality change: may become paranoid; shows definite personality change, provoking other people; may become restless and agitated; may pace and wander

Area of gait change: walks with short steps; has poor balance; loses motor and sensory control

Making the Diagnosis

The diagnosis of AD is one of the most difficult problems of the disease. The actual diagnosis depends on biopsies of brain tissue, which are not done while the person is alive. Therefore, the process of diagnosis requires a long time to rule out all the possible causes that might be treatable. Caution is essential to avoid making a misdiagnosis and labeling the individuals as irreversible and untreatable. The diagnosis is confirmed on autopsy. Findings on autopsy have been: atrophy of the brain; neurofibrillary tangles, senile plagues, or neurotic plagues; granulovacular bodies, which are changes in the brain cells showing fluid areas and granular material; and Hirano bodies, which encase ribosomes and keep protein bodies from forming (Figure 11.1 a-d).

It becomes very important for physicians to be able to know which clients can benefit from treatment and which clients cannot. On the following page are examples of primary irreversible diseases of dementia and examples of secondary reversible dementia.

Primary irreversible dementia: intellectual impairment which progresses from memory loss to total disability and is untreatable. *Examples:* Alzheimer's disease, multi-infarct dementia, Friedreich's ataxia, Huntington's disease, Parkinson's disease, Pick's disease, and Creutzfeldt–Jacob disease.

Secondary reversible dementia: intellectual impairment which is treatable and reversible. *Examples:* depression; stroke, minor; head injuries; infections; metabolic disorders (thyroid dysfunction, etc.); temporary (reversible) confusion, brought on by fluid imbalance, drugs, relocation, and so on.

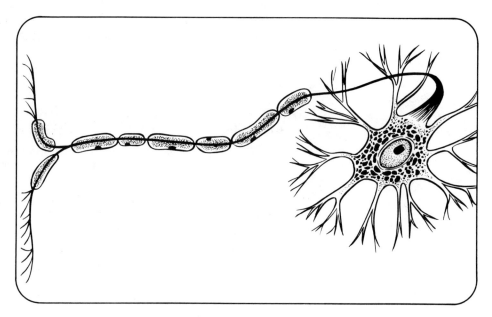

Figure 11.1(a). Normal neurons.

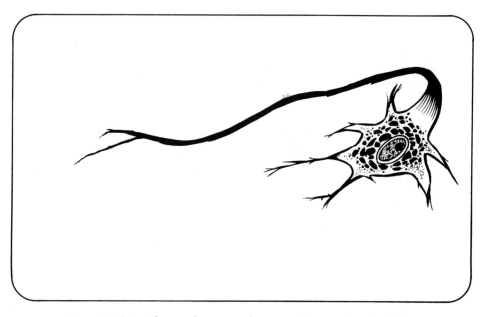

Figure 11.1(b). Abnormal neurons where neurofibers are in paired helix.

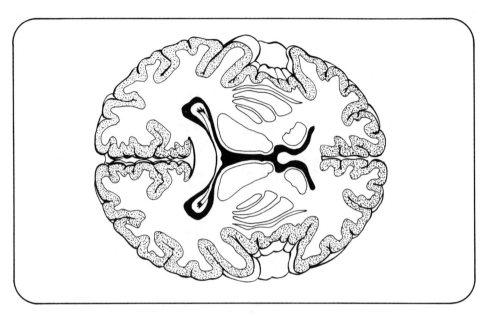

Figure 11.1(c). Normal brain section.

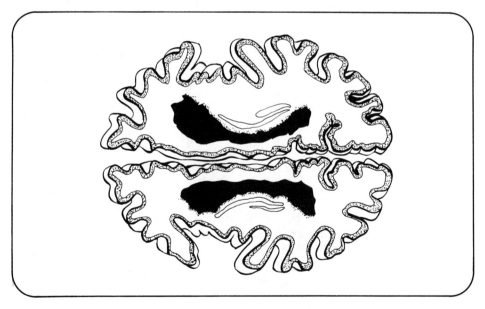

Figure 11.1(d). Brain section of patient with Alzheimer's disease.

Phases of Alzheimer's Disease

Following is a description of the four phases of Alzheimer's disease.

Phase	*Observable Behaviors*
1. *Forgetfulness.* Often this phase is insidious, develops slowly, and no one is quite sure that anything is wrong.	Less spontaneous, less sparkle; slower, less energy, less drive, less initiative; less discriminating; loss of words; slower to learn, slower to react; readily made angry; seeks and prefers the familiar, shuns the unfamiliar.
2. *Confusional, beginning.* While still functioning in many ways, the client may need supervision in specialized activities such as balancing a checkbook.	Much slower in speech and understanding; great difficulty in making decisions and plans; unable to calculate; increasingly self-absorbed; insensitive to feelings of others; avoids situations that may lead to failure; loses thread of a story.
3. *Confusional, advanced.* Now the client is obviously disabled.	Markedly changed behavior; uncertain as to how he or she is expected to act; directions need to be repeated; memory of recent past is poor or failing, memory of distant past astonishingly clear; loses orientation to time and place; invents words; misidentifies people; lethargic (lacks energy); little warmth in expressions.
4. *Dementia.* In this phase, help is needed with simple activities of daily living.	Apathetic (lacking feeling); poor remote or recent memory; cannot find the way around at all; difficulty with speech; no recognition of others: family, friends; hallucinations.

Reactions and Geriatric Nursing Assistant Responses

Sundowning syndrome   This term is derived from the behavior problems that occur in the evening.

Precipitating factors: May misinterpret surroundings; may want to go home; the environment is confusing; multiple stimuli result in the person's inability to cope; person may become agitated, more confused and anxious, and wants to wander; may call out to people in the family who are not there; may also be due to exhaustion and loneliness or to changes in sensory input (e.g., external sensory stimulation due to noises).

Suggested responses:

1. Provide for sufficient rest periods and alternate activity during the day.
2. Use touch reassurance if tolerated by client.

3. Provide familiar items to hold if client pulls at bedclothes.
4. Provide light so that shadows do not create false images.
5. Allow client to wander within observed area.
6. Provide a care giver familiar to client and make frequent checks on person's safety.
7. Follow communication techniques on checklists and guidelines.

Hallucinations This reaction is marked by seeing and hearing things for which there is no external stimulus. Can cause fear and anxiety—is a "real" situation for the person affected. Arguing or reasoning does not help. Communication that expresses understanding is necessary.

Suggested responses:

1. Use communication techniques on checklist and guidelines.
2. Provide reassurance; stay close by.
3. Do not argue or try to deny existence of stimulus.
4. Try calming techniques: back rub, warm milk.
5. Check skin if client complains of "bugs" and scratches.
6. Bring client to lighted area where personnel are nearby.
7. Inquire about client's vision and hearing checks to rule out physical causes.

Wandering This usually occurs with formerly active people; demented people seem to have an abundance of energy at times in the course of their disease. People who are physically active need a place for walking which provides for safety. Wandering requires evaluation: when, where, why of the wandering—the person may be looking for someone or something else of importance in his or her life. Outside wandering is of grave importance; people have died of overexposure or heart attack. A physical examination of each person is important; safety factors are also of grave importance (traffic, crime, etc.); may be subject to verbal/physical abuse.

Suggested responses:

1. Check to find out what needs or wants client has: food, fluids, toileting, and respond accordingly.
2. Assist client in finding own room.
3. Keep client busy if very restless.
4. If client wanders out of doors, follow in step and help to direct person back. (Do not grab and forcefully redirect.)
5. Check to be sure that identifying picture of resident is available in case client wanders beyond facility.
6. Provide exercise and safe place for walking without fear of leaving premises.

Agitation This reaction is marked by nervousness, restlessness, and/or worry in which the person exhibits anxiety. Person may not know the reason for it. May be due to changes in the brain, medications, environmental stimuli, sense of loss, or response to moods of others. Trying to respond with an explanation may not help. Reassurance and a calm affectionate response is helpful. Responding to the feeling of the person rather than the illogical concern provides the support needed.

Suggested responses:

1. Follow techniques of communication on checklist and guidelines.
2. Stay calm.
3. Reduce decision making by providing simple directions.
4. Try to find out what provokes agitation and plan to avoid those situations.
5. Try distractions that are soothing to client: music, singing, favorite story or item.

Delirium   This is sometimes called acute confusional state. There is a state of reduced level of consciousness causing disorientation, forgetfulness, with reduced ability to shift or focus attention; hallucinations may occur; sleepiness or wakefulness may occur in reverse time frame; increased or decreased motor activity; usually is a sudden change indicating a superimposed illness or medication reaction. Delirium requires investigation as to cause and treatment should be applied as quickly as possible.

Suggested responses:

1. Report sudden changes in behavior and any disorientation immediately to charge nurse.
2. Check vital signs and report findings to charge nurse.
3. Follow communication techniques on checklists and guidelines.
4. Provide frequent checks of client's condition.
5. Check client's intake and output for possible fluid imbalance, dehydration, or constipation.

Vocabulary Related to Cognitively Impaired People

The followiing terms are often used in describing cognitively impaired clients.

Acalculia: inability to do simple mathematical calculations.

Agnosia: inability to recognize familiar persons, places, things.

Aphasia: impaired communication in speech, writing, or signs due to dysfunction of brain centers in an affected hemisphere.

Apraxia: inability to perform purposeful movements when there is no paralysis or motor impairment.

Benign senescent forgetfulness (BSF): forgetfulness related to normal aging; related to diminished recall of details and not related to dementia.

Bulimia: abnormal sensation of hunger; abnormal appetite.

Catastrophic reactions: unusual response to a situation in which the person demonstrates a variety of reactions, such as: agitation, anger, pacing, wringing hands, paranoia, and violent striking out.

Delusions: false belief that are resistent to reason.

Dementia: loss or impairment of mental powers; loss of ability to remember, to function intellectually. Dementia is a group of symptoms, not the name of a disease.

Depression: state of lowered self-esteem with feelings of hopelessness and help-lessness; it can mimic dementia; it is treatable and reversible; often called a pseudodementia.

Dysphagia: impairment of speech; lack of coordination with failure to arrange words in proper order.

Dyspraxia: partial loss of ability to perform coordinated acts or movements.

Echolalia: repetition of meaningless words or sentences.

Hallucinations: seeing or hearing things without an external stimulus; visions or sounds do not exist.

Illusions: mistaken impression or interpretation that has a stimulus.

Perseveration: continued repetition of movement or words.

Pseudodementia: condition that mimics a true dementia but is treatable; such as depression.

Guidelines for Communication with the Cognitively Impaired

Verbal communication

1. Use short sentences and simple words.
2. Use reality orientation (see the checklist).
3. Avoid pronouns, use exact names (nouns) of persons/objects.
4. Provide one simple direction at a time.
5. Use the person's sensory language: for example, "I see"—use "imagine," "show," "look," and the like, which are of the same sense.
6. Always address the person by name and use your own name each time you communicate.
7. Avoid "many" care givers—restrict to as few people as possible when giving directions or eliciting feelings.
8. Use soft voice and unhurried style.

Nonverbal communication

1. Use eye contact at same level or from below level of person.
2. Do not use wild gestures.
3. Approach person from in front or from the side, not from the back.
4. Make gestures and facial expression agree with what is said.
5. Reduce external stimuli, noise especially.
6. Increase lighting in area if environment is dull.
7. Do not assume that the client does not have insight and understanding.
8. Use touch to convey affection, caring.

CHECKLIST FOR REALITY ORIENTATION

Equipment: Calendars with large days and numbers; clocks with large numbers; reality board giving date, day, weather, holiday, etc.; name tags on staff

	Yes	No
1. Face confused person and speak slowly and clearly.	—	—
2. Call person by name with each contact. Use the name he or she prefers.	—	—
3. State your name with each contact with person. Wear name tag.	—	—
4. State the day, date, and time during the day as appropriate.	—	—
5. Explain what you are going to do and why.	—	—
6. Give directions that are short and simple.	—	—
7. Refer to the clocks and calendars as appropriate.	—	—
8. Encourage the use and presence of familiar articles.	—	—
9. Discuss current events.	—	—
10. Encourage use of hearing aids and eyeglasses. Check to see if these items are of benefit when used.	—	—
11. Use touch in communicating when appropriate.	—	—
12. Be consistent, provide calm atmosphere, and try to reduce number of staff who have contact with confused person.	—	—
13. Maintain routines that reflect times of day; involve person in self-care as much as possible.	—	—
14. Maintain a familiar environment; do not rearrange furniture.	—	—
15. Observe person's activities and provide for safety.	—	—
16. Report and record person's progress with use of RO.	—	—

SKILL CHECKLIST FOR COMMUNICATION WITH THE COGNITIVELY IMPAIRED

	Yes	No
1. Use simple sentences.	—	—
2. Maintain eye contact.	—	—
3. Avoid multiple directions and choices.	—	—
4. Use facial expressions and gestures that agree with spoken words.	—	—
5. Avoid wild gestures.	—	—
6. Use appropriate tone of voice.	—	—
7. Convey respect and dignity.	—	—
8. Use touch with a caring manner.	—	—
9. Eliminate excessive external stimuli.	—	—
10. Use calm approach in attempts to understand responses.	—	—
11. Rephrase to assure understanding of what was said.	—	—
12. Respond to feelings of the impaired person.	—	—
13. Give praise where appropriate.	—	—
14. Provide for security and assurance of worth and dignity.	—	—
15. Provide time for person to respond or make other attempts to renew communication later.	—	—

Impact on the Cognitively Impaired Person and Family Members

The afflicted person   The aging person who is becoming or is cognitively impaired is experiencing a double insult; sensory deficits are occurring, including decreased hearing, vision, and touch; at the same time there is a decline in intellectual functioning. The afflicted person has a tremendous loss in self-esteem. As the client loses the ability to remember, to calculate a bank balance, pay bills, and drive a car, a sense of autonomy and independence is lost. The impact on the afflicted person is devastating and continues until he or she loses the ability to understand what is happening.

The family members   As the afflicted person becomes increasingly demented, role changes of family members occur. If the parent is the afflicted person, adult children assume the role of decision maker and take on parental responsibilities. Grief is constant for the adult child as the parent loses the ability to make decisions, undergoes a personality change, and seems to become someone totally different. The adult child becomes a care giver and may feel overloaded with responsibilities for his or her own family, job, and care-giving responsibilities. Family members often feel trapped and soon develop feelings of despair, anger, and frustration, intermingled with guilt for "not doing enough" for a beloved parent. If the afflicted person is a spouse, the other spouse feels the additional loss of a partner, a confidante, a loved one. He or she may assume the care giver role and takes on all the feelings described above as those of adult children. The household routine declines in both instances. Often there is a loss of social contact for the family if the afflicted person remains at home. Many friends do not understand the changes in the afflicted person and stay away. There is an increase in the financial burden since medical care increases for the afflicted person. Medicare does not cover the costs, and long-term care insurance is still unavailable for most families who find themselves in this situation.

Nursing Responses for Family Members and Client When Client Has Alzheimer's Disease

Phase	*Nursing Goals*	*Nursing Responses*
1. Forgetfulness	Client usually lives with family; maintain optimal self-care of client.	Encourage family to promote self-care of client; find support group and resources for family; begin reorientation reality therapy for client; encourage socialization and routines of daily living for client; keep familiar objects in same place.
2. Confusional, beginning	Family may need respite service; family continue with support group; family seek out resources; continue reality orientation for client.	Encourage client's self-care; provide outlet by listening to family members; encourage only one or few health care providers; establish trusting relationships with client and family members.

Responses for phases 1 and 2 apply if the client is at home or in the nursing home.

3. Confusional, advanced	Meet changing physical and emotional needs of resident and emotional needs of resident and family.	Monitor nutritional and fluid intake; provide for incontinence; protect from environment; monitor wandering; provide safety precautions; share responsibility with staff.
4. Dementia	Meet physical and emotional needs of resident and family; allow for grieving and loss—listen to family members; provide comfort measures to resident.	Speak in short sentences with simple directions to resident; avoid long explanations; avoid reality orientation unless it still helps; provide close observation; encourage family pictures and familiar items; reminisce with the resident

The client will more than likely be in a nursing home during stages 3 and 4.

RELATED DISORDERS

Disorders that have symptoms similar to Alzheimer's disease and lead to mental impairment and dementia are: multi-infarct dementia (MID), caused by many small strokes; Pick's disease; and Parkinson's dementia. There is no cure for these diseases; however, there are medications that help with symptoms. Medications are prescribed by the physician to ease the effects of deteriorating brain tissue. The goals of nursing care are to provide a safe, comfortable environment and to help the clients live life as independently as possible. The guidelines and checklists for geriatric nursing assistants apply to these clients just as they do for residents with Alzheimer's disease.

Notes about the Confused Resident

Giving a label of confusion to a resident is often done readily by health care workers when they find it difficult to manage the behavior of a resident in a nursing home. Once a label of confusion is given, it can affect the resident's quality of life. Too frequently, the person with the "confused" label is treated with less worth and the deserving sense of dignity is lost.

Before making a statement that a resident is confused, the following considerations are in order:

1. Observe all behaviors to ascertain if the "confusion" is isolated or displays disorientation as to time, place, object, purpose, and so on, after reality orientation is provided.
2. Determine if the resident thinks the behavior is inappropriate; compare with former behavior observed by staff or family members. It may very well be that the "confused" behavior is natural behavior for this particular resident.
3. Determine how you as a staff person perceive the resident. People who are considered less acceptable in appearance and socially undesirable are more readily considered confused compared to the resident who is considered more

likable. Ignoring the confused behavior and concentrating on the care needed may result in improved behavior and activities which come closer to what is expected.

Guidelines for Geriatric Nursing Assistants Who Work with Confused Residents

1. Work with the person, to indicate respect and foster dignity.
2. Be open to receive information; it helps to know that someone is listening.
3. Use rewards to strengthen desired behavior: eye contact, touch, smiles, praise.
4. Give choices when possible; encourage independence rather than perfection.
5. Work at a consistent, even pace with regular routine.
6. Follow through with what you say, never threaten, and avoid making promises.
7. Ignore performance failures.
8. Interpret or correct information when person is unsure about the environment and people in it.
9. Provide reality orientation around the clock, on all shifts.

Notes about the Depressed Resident

Older people in nursing homes may withdraw and appear to have no energy to participate in activities. A condition of pseudodementia or depression may be developing. Pseudodementia means resembling dementia, but it is reversible and treatable. Features that help to distinguish between pseudodementia and true dementia are listed in Figure 11.2. Residents with a depression can be helped if discovered in time and treatment and nursing responses are put into action. Sometimes medication is necessary, at least at the beginning of treatment.

	Depression Pseudodementia	True Dementia
The onset of the symptoms can be determined by the date	Usually	Not usually
Family is aware of the change in behavior	Usually	Not always
Resident has a history of some mental disorder	Usually	Not usually
Resident complains	Usually	Varies
Resident's effort to do tasks	Small	Great
Resident's emotional reaction	Great distress	Varies (often concealed)
Resident lacks social skills	Early	Late
Resident's attention and concentration	Good	Poor

Figure 11.2. Comparison of depression pseudodementia and true dementia.

Geriatric nursing assistant responses for residents who are depressed

1. Report any changes of behavior that lead to withdrawal to the charge nurse.
2. Check on what situations cause resident to become sad and withdrawn.
3. Spend special time with the resident indicating that he or she is worthy and valued.
4. Provide reassurance that you and the staff care.
5. Encourage the resident to talk. This may take some time. Just being there and offering touch or other appropriate nonverbal behavior may bring about conversation.
6. Provide a volunteer to work with resident on a simple task. Have same person return on a routine basis. Perhaps a bond will begin to grow and the volunteer can help the resident rejoin in activities and socialization. Provide ongoing support and encouragement to the volunteer.

Suicide among the Elderly

The suicide rate among the elderly is considered high and is expected to increase. In her book *Nursing and the Aged*, Irene Burnside stated that suicide rates increased for people over age 75. "At ages 75 and over, suicide rates rose 8 percent" (*Statistical Bulletin*, 1982, p. 712). Men are three times more likely to commit suicide than women. By the age of 85 the ratio of male suicides to women is 12:1. Factors that have been found to place the elderly at high risk for suicide include: being male, living alone, poor health, retirement or out of work, loneliness, low self-esteem, history of poor relationships, and a poor marital history. Depression often occurs prior to suicidal attempts. The individual who contemplates suicide will make comments which reflect despair and hopelessness and a wish to be dead.

Geriatric nursing assistant responses for persons who are suicidal

1. Report to the charge nurse any sign of depression or expression of despair, or attempt to end one's life. Mental health professionals can be contacted.
2. Listen to the person's expressions nonjudgmentally.
3. Try to determine who and what is meaningful in the person's life and provide contacts and activities to reinforce the importance of involvement with the person or activities.
4. Provide frequent attention to the person and work with the mental health consultants as part of the health care team.
5. Provide a warm, sensitive, caring attitude when attending an elderly person who is showing signs of low self-esteem and despair.

KEY POINTS

1. The cognitively impaired person may have Alzheimer's disease or a related disorder. It is estimated approximately 50 percent of nursing home residents have progressive cognitive impairment.
2. Some clients with apparent cognitive impairment may be treatable and reversible. Sudden changes in a person's behavior should be reported immediately.

3. The diagnosis of an untreatable dementia is difficult and requires extensive testing by the physician.
4. There are specific nursing assistant responses that the geriatric nursing assistant can apply to ease the discomforts and confusion experienced by the cognitively impaired person and his or her family members.
5. Effective communication techniques applied to cognitively impaired residents may help to comfort the resident experiencing hallucinations, agitation, or other catastrophic reactions.
6. Reporting behavior changes indicating confusion, depression, or potential suicidal behavior of residents may prevent an irreversible dementia and/or a suicide.
7. Caring for the cognitively impaired resident is one of the most challenging situations the geriatric nursing assistant will encounter.

SELF-CHECK

True or False. Place a T in front of statements that are true, an F in front of statements that are false.

_____ 1. Alzheimer's disease is a secondary dementia.
_____ 2. The diagnosis of Alzheimer's is relatively easy.
_____ 3. Family members of Alzheimer's victims need as much help as the Alzheimer victim.
_____ 4. Sundowning syndrome occurs toward morning.
_____ 5. Delirium means dreaming.
_____ 6. Pseudodementia and confusion may be related to Alzheimer's disease.
_____ 7. It is best to use large gestures when speaking to demented residents.
_____ 8. It is best to approach the demented person from the front or side when communicating.
_____ 9. The depressed resident may be treatable.
_____ 10. The confused resident can be mistaken as untreatable.
_____ 11. More elderly women than men commit suicide.

Provide a list of five nursing responses for the following residents.

12. Mr. Hall, a 65-year-old gentleman with second-stage symptoms of AD, has been forgetting things lately, and then he begins to try to cover up the fact. He is always asking if it is time to eat when he just finished eating. His family is embarrassed when he does this and they try to get him to be quiet. This seems to agitate Mr. Hall. What can you do?

13. Mrs. Stonewall is 75 years old and has lived in the nursing home for about a year. Her husband passed away 3 weeks ago. She always goes to Bingo on Tuesday afternoon, but for the last 2 weeks she has been staying in her room. She has started asking to have her meals in her room. She rarely smiles anymore. What may be happening? What will you do?

14. Mr. Brown is 80 years old. He has lived alone most of his life, having had several broken marriages. He has been heard saying, "I am ready to give it up." He has been giving his personal possessions away to other residents. He has started to stay in his room staring out the window. What are your next responses? What risk factors is Mr. Brown exhibiting?

SUGGESTED ACTIVITIES

1. Invite a member from the Alzheimer disease support group to talk to the class about the challenges he/she faces as a care giver to a loved one with Alzheimer's disease.
2. Talk with family members who visit Alzheimer residents where you work. Ask about their reactions to the changes they see in the resident and how they feel about the client being in the nursing home.
3. Visit a special unit for Alzheimer residents and compare the environment with the environment of other units. Find out what nursing responses they provide.

CLINICAL APPLICATION

Using the problem-solving worksheet provided at the end of this unit, select a cognitively impaired person with Alzheimer's disease or a related disorder and outline implications for care of the person and geriatric nursing assistant responses for family members.

Cerebral Vascular Accidents: Age-Related Changes

TERMINAL PERFORMANCE OBJECTIVE

Given information on cerebral vascular accidents and appropriate geriatric nursing assistant responses, be able to provide geriatric nursing assistant responses to clients who have had a cerebral vascular accident.

Enabling Objectives

1. Define cerebral vascular accident and identify its medical abbreviation.
2. Define contributing causes: thrombus, embolus, arteriosclerosis, and hypertension.
3. Describe five physical changes to be expected in a person with a cerebral vascular accident.
4. Describe three emotional changes to be expected in a person with a cerebral vascular accident.
5. Identify geriatric nursing assistant responses for clients with cerebral vascular accidents.

6. Provide nursing assistant responses to clients who experience cerebral vascular accidents.

REVIEW SECTION

The topics the geriatric nursing assistant should review with the instructor are the changes that occur in the nervous and circulatory systems as aging occurs.

PHYSICAL CHANGES DUE TO CVA

The common name for a cerebral vascular accident (CVA) is stroke. A stroke is a condition that is caused by changes in circulation to brain tissue. These changes may be due to: formation of a blood clot in a vessel which obstructs flow of blood (thrombus) either completely or partially; a ruptured blood vessel due to weakening of the vessel wall (aneurysm); or a part of a thrombus that breaks off and interrupts brain circulation (embolus) (Figure 11.3).

Conditions such as atherosclerosis (hardening of the inner lining of arteries) and hypertension (high blood pressure) contribute to stroke and have an increasing tendency to occur in older people. Strokes occur suddenly in varying degree: Some may be quite severe and involve major vessels to the brain; other strokes are less severe and may result in ministrokes, known as transient ischemic attacks (TIAs). The severe stroke is an acute condition causing loss of consciousness, difficult respirations, and paralysis of one side of the body. The blood pressure is usually elevated and body temperature may be quite high (106 °F or above).

Damage to the right side of the brain may result in left-sided paralysis. Damage to the left side of the brain may result in right-sided paralysis (in the following pages we provide more detailed signs and functions disturbed by stroke). Knowing what kind of damage has occurred to the nervous system helps the geriatric nursing assistant to anticipate what nursing measures may be needed. When damage does occur to brain tissue, the afflicted person suffers many emotional as well as physical changes.

EMOTIONAL CHANGES DUE TO CVA

Emotional changes occur due to disturbance in the parts of the brain that involve emotional control. The sudden inability to perform routine tasks adds frustration to an altered emotional condition. Emotional outbursts of tears or laughter are not uncommon. The care giver must be very patient and tactful and not add to the individual's embarrassment by showing disapproval. A loss in self-esteem and sense of worth are also common.

The person with left-sided brain damage may experience a condition called *aphasia*. Aphasia is loss or impairment of the capacity to use words. Aphasia may take different forms. Some people may understand what is said but cannot respond correctly (expressive aphasia). Other people cannot understand words and cannot express themselves (global aphasia). Other people can say certain words but say them incorrectly and at the wrong time. The speech therapist is a professional who can be of great help to persons with aphasia and a valuable member of the care team. The geriatric nursing assistant can learn how to continue to respond to the aphasic person by following recommendations from the

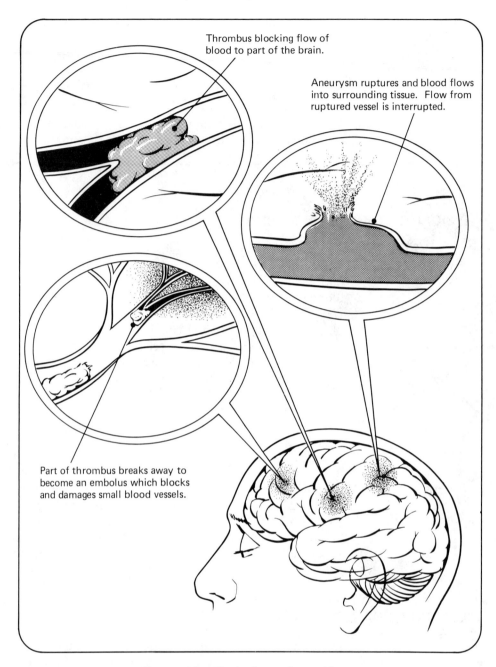

Thrombus blocking flow of blood to part of the brain.

Aneurysm ruptures and blood flows into surrounding tissue. Flow from ruptured vessel is interrupted.

Part of thrombus breaks away to become an embolus which blocks and damages small blood vessels.

Figure 11.3. Cerebral vascular accidents.

speech therapist. Everyone on the care team should follow these recommendations around the clock.

Nursing care of a person with a stroke is very challenging. The holistic philosophy of care with the purpose of helping the person to achieve maximum potential in daily independent living should be the guide for all care givers.

Geriatric Nursing Assistant Responses

The following list of nursing responses should be considered for residents who suffer a cerebral vascular accident.

1. Provide proper positioning and body alignment while the person is in bed and when up in a wheelchair.
2. Follow recommendations from the physical therapist when providing range-of-motion exercises, transfer techniques, and use of adaptive devices. Adaptive devices include splints for limb positioning to prevent or correct deformities; modified utensils when eating; and equipment to assist in daily dressing. See figures 11.4, 11.5, and 11.6.
3. Provide for daily bathing and skin care: back rubs, lotion to potential pressure areas, protection from decubiti formation when in bed and in a wheelchair.
4. Encourage deep breathing and coughing.
5. Assist with feeding and adequate fluid intake. A special feeding plan may be necessary if a resident has difficulty eating and swallowing.
6. Monitor urinary output. An indwelling catheter may be needed if bladder control is affected; however, it should be only temporary and bladder retraining started as soon as possible.

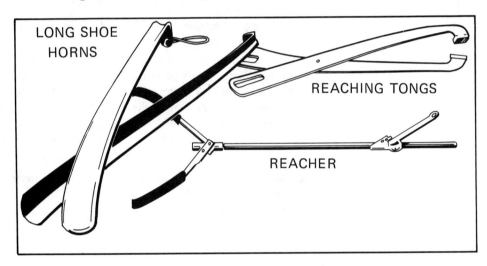

Figure 11.4. Adaptive devices.

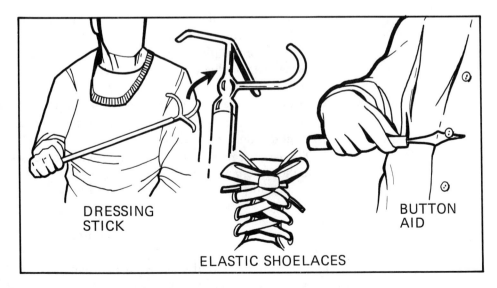

Figure 11.5. Adaptive devices.

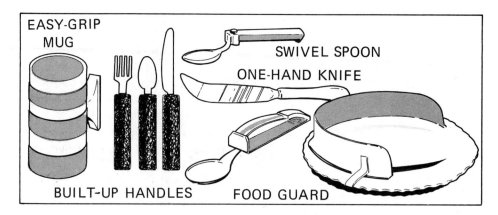

Figure 11.6.   Adaptive devices.

7. Blood pressure readings may be taken throughout the day to monitor any hypertension.

8. Apply support restraints (as ordered) to help resident maintain proper body position when out of bed.

9. Establish a communication system if speech is impaired. Use flash cards with pictures of key words or put cards on a communication board. All speech should be confined to simple sentences and single concepts. When giving directions, give one simple direction at a time. Approach person from unaffected side. Sometimes stroke victims can see from only one side. Vision from affected side may be lost or diminished.

10. Provide emotional support with a positive attitude.

11. Reduce the number of care givers in order to increase consistency of care and to eliminate distractions.

12. Gradually help person to do self-care; start with small tasks and increase as much as resident can tolerate.

KEY POINTS

1. A cerebral vascular accident (CVA) occurs suddenly and may cause temporary or longer-lasting loss of function.

2. Known contributing causes of CVAs are related to changes that often occur with aging: hypertension, atherosclerosis, formation of a thrombus, embolus, or aneurysm.

3. Physical changes resulting from strokes include paralysis and aphasia.

4. Emotional changes resulting from strokes include outbursts of crying, laughter, and frustration.

5. The geriatric nursing assistant can provide responses to meet all dimensions of the person, with the goal of helping the afflicted resident in reaching his/her maximum potential for independent living.

SELF-CHECK

1. Mr. Brown has told you he has had many strokes but that he was never paralyzed. What kind of stroke might he be referring to, and what is the medical abbreviation?

2. Mrs. Jones has aphasia. She is trying to learn to say the right word. How can you help her?

3. Describe three underlying changes that accompany the aging process that contribute to CVAs.

4. Mr. Black had a stroke 6 months ago. He has periods of crying without any apparent cause. What can you do to help?

5. Mrs. Kelly has some paralysis of her right side. She is learning to feed herself with her left hand. What devices might help her? How will you transfer her into a wheelchair?

SUGGESTED ACTIVITIES

1. Visit a meeting of a local Stroke Club to learn how the members have adjusted to their lives.
2. Talk with some of the residents who have had strokes to learn of their feelings about themselves and their care.
3. Visit a rehabilitation department to find out about the procedures they follow to help stroke patients to rehabilitate.

CLINICAL APPLICATION

Using the problem-solving worksheet provided at the end of this unit, select a resident with a stroke and provide geriatric nursing assistant responses.

Diabetes Mellitus: Age-Related Changes

TERMINAL PERFORMANCE OBJECTIVE

Given information on diabetes mellitus and geriatric nursing assistant responses, be able to provide nursing assistant responses to a resident with diabetes mellitus.

Enabling Objectives

1. Define diabetes mellitus.
2. Distinguish between hypoglycemia and hyperglycemia.
3. Distinguish between the signs and symptoms of diabetic shock and diabetic coma.
4. Identify nursing assistant responses for residents who have diabetes mellitus.
5. Apply nursing assistant responses to residents with diabetes mellitus.

REVIEW SECTION

The topics the geriatric nursing assistant should review with the instructor are the endocrine system, functions of the pancreas, and the usual glucose urine testing procedures for residents with diabetes mellitus.

THE DISEASE AND ITS COURSE

Diabetes mellitus is a disease characterized by insufficient insulin and failure of body cells to utilize glucose resulting in hyperglycemia, too much sugar in the blood. Studies have shown that with increasing age, there is a decline in the body's tolerance of glucose as well as a decrease in the production of insulin. Another factor that is conducive to elderly people developing diabetes is the reduction in physical activity, which normally helps to utilize glucose for energy. Since there is usually less activity for the older person, and if that person continues to eat many carbohydrates, there is more tendency to accumulate glucose, the end product of carbohydrate metabolism in the bloodstream.

The kind of diabetes that is diagnosed in elderly people is called type II. This type develops in later years and is usually controlled without the need for insulin. The doctor usually orders an oral medication and special diabetic diet with reduced carbohydrates.

Type I diabetes is referred to as the juvenile type because of its early onset; it does require that the person receive insulin. Type I diabetes can be very severe and leads to serious complications over a long period of time. The diabetic diet is part of the treatment for both type I and type II diabetes.

TREATMENT

When caring for the diabetic who receives insulin, there are several important considerations (Figure 11.7). If the person receives too much insulin or does not eat portions of the diet, a condition known as insulin shock can occur. Insulin shock is brought on by hypoglycemia, too little glucose in the blood. The opposite condition of insulin shock is diabetic coma. In this instance, there is not enough insulin and too much glucose in the blood. Figure 11.8 shows the difference in the two conditions.

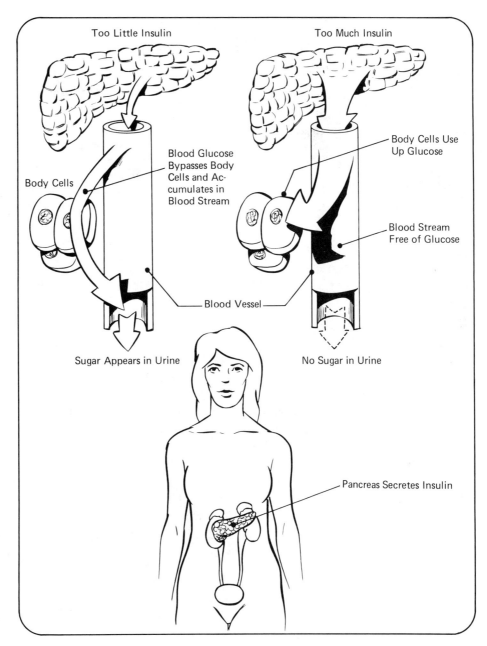

Figure 11.7. Insulin reaction.

The geriatric nursing assistant, upon recognizing the signs and symptoms of either condition, must report these immediately to the charge nurse. The person in diabetic coma will require insulin intravenously. The person in insulin shock will require carbohydrates immediately. Usually orange juice, candy, or sometimes glucose intravenously must be given.

Diabetes of long duration leads to complications. The arteries of diabetics often become blocked so badly, especially in the feet, that amputation may become the only alternative. Blindness, due to damage of the retina, may result. Cataracts, hypertension, and nerve damage, especially of the extremities, are common with long-term diabetics. Tingling and numbness can occur in the fingers and toes. Temperature changes are difficult to determine.

	Diabetic Insulin Shock (Hypoglycemia)	Diabetic Coma (Hyperglycemia)
Possible causes	Too much insulin	Too little insulin
	Excessive exercise activity	Infection, vomiting, overeating
	Insufficient carbohydrate intake	
Onset	Sudden	Slow
Behavior	Irritable, excited, hungry	Sluggish
Skin	Cold, clammy, pale	Hot, dry, flushed
Breathing	About usual	Deep, fruity odor
Pulse	Rapid, thready	Normal to slower
Urine	No glucose, no acetone	Glucose present, acetone present
Response to treatment	Sugar given—fast	Insulin given—slow

Figure 11.8. Symptoms of insulin shock and diabetic coma.

Geriatric Nursing Assistant Responses

1. Monitor and report how much of what foods the diabetic does not eat. Report these to the charge nurse so that supplements may be given. Encourage eating of all foods served.
2. Assist with extra care to the feet: Watch for any signs of change—redness, paleness, tenderness, swelling, or any other signs of infection. Toenails must be trimmed carefully by licensed nurse, physician, or podiatrist. *Geriatric nursing assistants do not trim nails of diabetics.*
3. Encourage good-fitting shoes, sturdy but comfortable.
4. Provide for exercise; guard against excessive exercises.
5. Perform routine urine testing as ordered. Report results to charge nurse.
6. Report any changes in resident's condition which may indicate that an infection is starting: signs of a cold, diarrhea, nausea and vomiting, and inflammation of the skin. Any of these signs may be enough to cause an imbalance of the metabolism of carbohydrates and lead to complications.
7. Monitor temperature of bath or shower water of diabetics who lose sensitivity to hot and cold. Self-care diabetics can burn themselves in hot water and not realize it.

The elderly person with type II diabetes is less likely to develop severe reactions. The disease is often controlled with diet. The problems occur when additional stress is confronted by the elderly person. The stress factor could be a common cold. Therefore, the geriatric nursing assistant taking care of an elderly diabetic should be very observant of any changes and report them immediately.

KEY POINTS

1. Diabetes mellitus, type II, is more common with elderly people when there is insufficient insulin for utilization of glucose by body cells.
2. Two severe reactions that can occur are hypoglycemia seen in insulin shock, and hyperglycemia in diabetic coma.

3. The geriatric nursing assistant should be alert to any changes experienced by the diabetic client and report these immediately.

SELF-CHECK

1. Define diabetes mellitus.

2. *Hypoglycemia* means _____ and occurs when there is _____ insulin in the body.

3. *Hyperglycemia* means _____ and occurs when there is _____ insulin in the body.

4. Mr. Willis is 70 years old and has had diabetes for 45 years. He takes insulin every morning. He has not eaten his lunch today because he said he feels like he is getting a cold and isn't hungry. Answer the following questions.
   a. What should you do about this problem?

   b. What reaction might you expect? What symptoms would you watch for?

   c. If Mr. Willis has a Clinitest every day before meals, what result would you expect since he hasn't eaten since breakfast after he had insulin?

SUGGESTED ACTIVITIES

1. Practice testing of urine for sugar and acetone using the tests used in your facility. Become very familiar with the color charts and their interpretations. Practice charting the results.
2. Visit the American Diabetes Association office in your community to learn about their functions and the diabetic materials they have.
3. Invite a person with diabetes to class to discuss the disease and what it is like to give insulin to oneself every day.

CLINICAL APPLICATION

Using the problem-solving worksheet provided in this unit, select a person who has diabetes mellitus and provide geriatric nursing assistant responses.

Cancer: Age-Related Changes

TERMINAL PERFORMANCE OBJECTIVE

Given information on cancer and geriatric nursing assistant responses, be able to provide geriatric nursing assistant responses to a resident with cancer.

Enabling Objectives

1. Define the term *cancer* and identify the abbreviation used to designate it.
2. Identify five suspected causes of cancer.
3. Describe three modes of treatment for cancer.
4. Identify geriatric nursing assistant responses when caring for residents with cancer.
5. Apply geriatric nursing assistant responses to residents with cancer.

REVIEW SECTION

The topics the geriatric nursing assistant should review with the instructor are communications and the grieving process.

THE DISEASE AND ITS COURSE

The diagnosis of cancer has come to mean a dismal lifetime for some people. It is especially sad when a diagnosis is late in the progression of the disease. However, there are many people who have had an early diagnosis and, with treatment, were able to live happy lives. The geriatric nursing assistant can provide responses that help the person with cancer "live" with the disease and not "die" with it.

Cancer is a term taken from a Latin word meaning "crab." Cancer is a malignant tumor that can grow to unlimited dimensions and, in doing so, invades healthy tissue. Cancer spreads out like the crab does with its legs. The abbreviation CA is often used to refer to a cancerous condition. The spread of cancer from one part of the body to another is referred to as *metastasis*.

Cancer is considered a disease of aging; however, there are forms of cancer that afflict younger people. Tumors of the brain occur in young as well as old people. Leukemias also occur in childhood. With the exception of these, age is the single greatest factor in developing malignancy (another term used synonymously with "cancer"). Sixty percent of all cancers occur after 60 years of age. The incidence goes up to 1 in 10 people having a cancer by age 70. Reasons given for more older people developing cancer have been: accumulation of cancer-causing agents, and decreased efficiency of the immune system. Cancer of the lung is greatest in men, while breast cancer is the highest type of cancer for women. Colorectal cancer is fairly equal for men and women.

Cancer has also been called an "environmental disease." This means that our environment contains cancer-producing agents that we consume or with which we come in contact. Today, tobacco has been named as a serious contaminant to our bodies and has been definitely linked to lung cancer. Cigarette smoke has been linked to lung problems of people who do not smoke. No-smoking bans are becoming more prevalent in airplanes and public places because of the effects of cigarette smoke.

Other cancer-causing agents have been found in soil, fish, food, and water—all consumable. The lack of fiber in our diets has been associated with the increase in colorectal cancers. It has been noted that the highly processed food consumed in the United States causes delay of passage of feces. As a result, bacteria accumulate in the bowel and can cause cell changes that become precancerous. For some people, the precancerous tissue becomes cancerous.

TREATMENT

In general, how far the disease has progressed when diagnosed has a great deal to do with how long a person will live. Medical research has improved therapy and allowed many more people to continue to live longer than ever before.

Therapy takes three forms:

1. *Surgery.* The diseased part is removed.
2. *Radiation therapy.* X-rays or gamma rays are applied to a lesion from outside the body or by placing a radioactive isotope into tissues that are cancerous.
3. *Chemotherapy.* Anticancer drugs are introduced by intravenous route, by intramuscular route, or by mouth.

The therapy can be very disturbing to patients because of the side effects. Some people elect not to have any therapy because of these side effects. Surgery is usually the least damaging because, once the surgical site has healed, there are few aftereffects. This is not true of radiation or chemotherapy, which take from weeks to months to complete.

The side effects of radiation may be: damage to healthy cells, fatigue, loss of appetite, vomiting, diarrhea, and frequent urination. Some skin damage may also result, as well as a drop in the red blood cell count.

The side effects of chemotherapy may be: nausea, vomiting, loss of appetite, loss of hair over the entire body, severe inflammation of the gums (stomatitis), constipation, tingling and numbness in the legs, and depression of blood-forming organs. There may be accompanying fatigue, and abnormal bleeding from mucous membranes.

The part of the body affected will determine specific nursing measures to be given. In general, the geriatric nursing assistant should adopt a sensitive attitude and use abilities to listen and to allow for the expression of feelings that the resident will have. The resident who has cancer may already have had a series of treatments which helped to ease symptoms. The cancer patient may be in the nursing home because it is simply a matter of time before the disease overwhelms the body's ability to defend itself. A positive, caring attitude is essential for all care givers.

Geriatric Nursing Assistant Responses

In caring for cancer patients, the geriatric nursing assistant must know what kind of treatment the resident is receiving and then be on the alert for what responses will be needed.

1. Nutritional snacks should be provided when a resident has a loss of appetite. Snacks should be available regardless of time of day or night.
2. If resident is undergoing therapy, the nurses at the place of treatment may have some good suggestions for nutritional supplements. Ask that they be contacted.
3. Provide a pleasant eating time.
4. Suggest (if permitted) that family members bring in a favorite food.
5. Communicate with family members to help them express feelings.
6. Provide personal care with attention to the skin. Note any skin changes and report immediately.
7. Monitor bowel movements for any diarrhea or constipation. Report immediately.
8. Report any nausea or vomiting immediately.
9. Provide mouth care frequently.
10. Report any pain immediately (note what kind of pain and where it is).
11. Suggest a head covering, such as a wig, to cover lost hair.
12. Be a sensitive and empathetic care giver. Listen and promote self-expression of residents who are living with cancer.

KEY POINTS

1. Cancer can be a diagnosis that produces many different responses in people.
2. How late the diagnosis is made will partially determine a person's length of life.
3. Surgery, radiation, and chemotherapy remain the usual forms of treatment.
4. Therapy can have some side effects that may cause much discomfort.
5. The geriatric nursing assistant can be a positive, sensitive care giver and help the afflicted person "live" with cancer.

SELF-CHECK

1. Define cancer and write an acceptable abbreviation.

2. Explain the phrase: "Cancer is an environmental disease."

3. What are the usual modes of cancer treatment?

4. Mrs. Rose is 80 years old and dying from breast cancer. Some days she eats fairly well, but other days she barely eats at all. Her family visits daily. Mrs. Rose refused all forms of treatment. List at least five nursing assistant responses for Mrs. Rose and her family.

SUGGESTED ACTIVITIES

1. Visit the local cancer society to learn what activities they do to support cancer patients.
2. Invite a person who has cancer to class to talk about his/her treatment and effects of treatment.

CLINICAL APPLICATION

Using the problem-solving worksheet provided at the end of this unit, select a resident with cancer and provide geriatric nursing assistant responses.

Arthritis: Age-Related Changes

TERMINAL PERFORMANCE OBJECTIVE

Given information on arthritis and geriatric nursing assistant responses, be able to apply geriatric nursing assistant responses to a resident with arthritis.

Enabling Objectives

1. Define arthritis.
2. Differentiate between rheumatoid and osteoarthritis.
3. Identify nursing assistant responses for care of arthritic residents.
4. Apply geriatric nursing assistant responses to residents with arthritis.

REVIEW SECTION

The topics the nursing assistant should review with the nursing instructor are the musculoskeletal system and age-related changes.

THE DISEASE AND ITS COURSE

Arthritis can be a symptom or a disease. *Arthritis* means inflammation of a joint. *Osteoarthritis* is a degenerative joint disease which causes more crippling of older adults than does any other disease. About 40 million Americans, including 85 to 90 percent of those over 65 years of age, have some changes in weight-bearing joints involved in osteoarthritis. Osteoarthritis is chiefly a disease of cartilage degeneration (Figure 11.9).

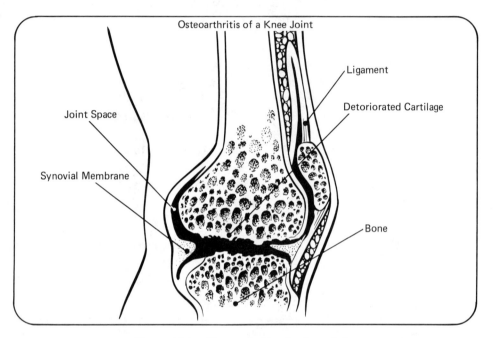

Figure 11.9. Osteoarthritis of a knee joint.

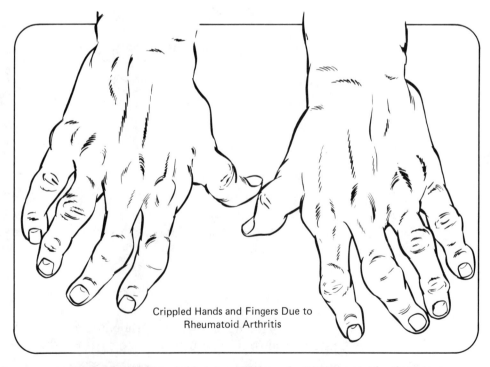

Figure 11.10. Crippled hands and fingers due to rheumatoid arthritis.

Rheumatoid arthritis is a systemic disease (relates to a system). This type of arthritis is associated with other immunological diseases. Rheumatoid arthritis affects the young, starting around the late third or fourth decade of life, but also appears late in life. In fact, the presence increases as people age. Rheumatoid arthritis causes crippling and deformity of joints (Figure 11.10).

Both osteoarthritis and rheumatoid arthritis cause pain, joint limitation of motion, stiffness, and swelling. The specific cause for either disease is unknown. A comparison of the two types of arthritis is shown in Figure 11.11.

Osteoarthritis (OA)	Rheumatoid Arthritis (RA)
Involves weight-bearing joints: hips, knees, and lumbar spine	Involves wrists, feet, especially joints of toes and fingers, also involves knees and shoulders
All joints may show some degeneration	Joints involved are usually symmetrical (both sides) of body; is considered an inflammatory arthritis
Is considered a noninflammatory type of arthritis	Acute flare-ups occur with redness, swelling, and severe pain followed by periods of remission
Deterioration is in the cartilage; pain increases with joint deterioration	Deterioration is primarily in the synovial lining; pain increases as joints deteriorate
Less observable deformity of joints	Severe deformity of joints
Common to all people	More common to women than men

Figure 11.11.   A comparison between osteoarthritis and rheumatoid arthritis.

TREATMENT

Treatment of the person with either type of arthritis involves four phases: education about the disease, physical therapy, drug therapy, and surgical joint replacement if selected by the client. People with joint disease must learn how to care for themselves and what to expect. The physical therapist helps to establish an individualized exercise routine and treatment schedule. Treatments may include warm water baths (Figure 11.12), paraffin baths (Figure 11.13), and range-of-motion exercises using exercise apparatus. The balance of exercise and activity becomes important. Lack of exercise may hasten joint stiffness and development of contractures with a resulting permanent deformity. On the other hand, joint pain may be severe enough that the client will not want to exercise.

Drug therapy helps to relieve the pain in both forms of arthritis and to lessen the inflammatory process of rheumatoid arthritis. Surgery may be recommended when joints become so deteriorated that exercise and mobility are difficult. Inactivity leads to many complications that result in the decline of the person's ability to function.

Geriatric Nursing Assistant Responses

The ultimate goal of nursing care is to assist the resident to function as independently as possible.

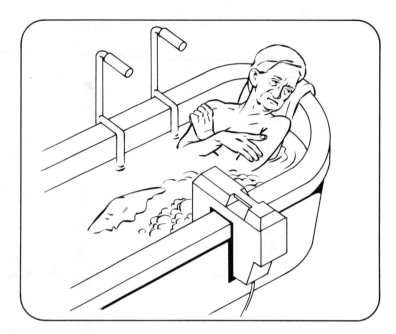

Figure 11.12.   Whirlpool bathtub. Warm baths aid the person with arthritis in exercising joints.

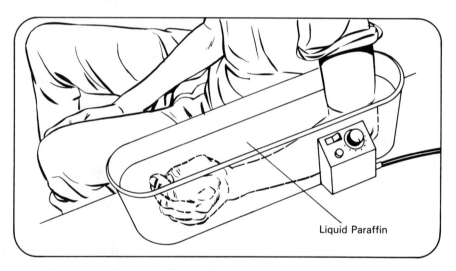

Liquid Paraffin

Figure 11.13   Paraffin tub for coating fingers, hands, and lower arms. Paraffin is warm and provides a warm, protective coating which holds heat to joints.

1. Report any pain immediately: Be able to identify type and location and follow through to be sure that pain is relieved.
2. Report any indication of acute arthritic reaction—joint swelling, redness, motion limitation, fever, warmth of the joint.
3. Carry out range-of-motion exercises as prescribed.
4. Apply prescribed corrective devices to support limbs that are deformed.
5. Assist resident to maintain posture. This may require restraining devices, which must be ordered by the doctor.
6. Provide adaptive eating and dressing utensils so that the resident can be as independent as possible.

7. Provide for rest periods.
8. Encourage socialization and participation in activities that help to distract resident from self-centering.
9. Help resident to learn about his or her condition. Provide time to listen and direct questions to appropriate care team members.
10. Help to create an atmosphere of improvement. Give praise for each step of progress.

KEY POINTS

1. Arthritis can be a symptom of disease or a disease in itself.
2. There are two types of arthritis fairly common with aging people: osteoarthritis and rheumatoid arthritis.
3. Most people over 65 years of age show some degenerative joint change.
4. The goal of the geriatric nursing assistant's responses is to assist the arthritic resident to be functioning as independently as possible.

SELF-CHECK

1. Arthritis is inflammation of _____ .
2. Osteoarthritis differs from rheumatoid arthritis in what three ways?

3. Mrs. Smith has severe joint deformity of her hands and toes. She requires corrective shoes and tries to walk with a walker. She is right-handed but has great difficulty in cutting meats, holding a glass, and using a fork. What nursing assistant measures can you provide to increase her functioning at an independent level?

SUGGESTED ACTIVITIES

1. Visit the Arthritis Foundation to learn what activities they have to help people with arthritis.
2. Speak to a hospital surgical team member to learn of the newest procedures to correct joint deformities.
3. Visit a rehabilitation center to learn what kinds of therapy are recommended to arthritic patients.

CLINICAL APPLICATION

Using the problem-solving worksheet provided at the end of this unit, select a resident with arthritis and provide geriatric nursing assistant responses.

Chronic Obstructive Pulmonary Disease: Age-Related Changes

TERMINAL PERFORMANCE OBJECTIVE

Given information about the chronic obstructive diseases of the lung and appropriate geriatric nursing assistant responses, be able to provide geriatric nursing assistant responses to residents with chronic obstructive pulmonary disease.

Enabling Objectives

1. Define chronic obstructive pulmonary disease and the acceptable medical abbreviation.
2. Explain the differences between asthma, emphysema, and bronchitis.
3. Identify nursing assistant responses for residents with chronic obstructive pulmonary disease.
4. Apply geriatric nursing assistant responses to residents with chronic obstructive pulmonary disease.

REVIEW SECTION

The topics the geriatric nursing assistant should review with the instructor are the age-related changes in the pulmonary system, the postural drainage procedures, and oxygen safety.

THE DISEASE AND ITS COURSE

Chronic obstructive pulmonary disease (COPD) is really a combination of diseases which are difficult to differentiate in the elderly person. The elderly person with COPD usually has symptoms that relate to all three diseases: coughing, wheezing, frequent upper respiratory infections, and shortness or difficulty with breathing (dyspnea).

There are changes in the lungs which accompany aging that result in decreased functional ability. There is less gas exchanged and less lung tissue. The strength of respiratory muscles is weakened. The thoracic cage becomes more rigid. The lung tissue is less elastic. There is also a weakness in the pulmonary defense mechanisms against accumulation of secretion and aspiration which might contribute to the frequency of lung infections in older people.

Smoking for a period of years certainly has had greatly damaging effects on lung tissue. Smoking is known to decrease resistance to disease by weakening the function of the hair-like cilia that help to move foreign agents up and out of the bronchial tree. Smoking has a tendency to make the cilia immobile, therefore giving minute foreign material the opportunity to move into pulmonary passage ways. The changes related to aging and a history of smoking contribute to the occurrence of lung diseases among the elderly. The three diseases involved in COPD are asthma, emphysema, and chronic bronchitis (Figure 11.14).

Asthma is a chronic disease that results from a sensitivity of the trachea and bronchi to many types of stimuli. The bronchi become spasmatic and the free flow of oxygen in and carbon dioxide out of the lungs becomes difficult. Mucous secretions become excessive. Asthma can start in childhood or later in life. Some stimulants that may cause an attack are: viral infections, smoke, cold air, and polluted air. Treatment is directed at reversing the bronchial spasms to allow a free exchange of air. Medications by mouth or by inhalation are usually ordered, which help the bronchi to dilate.

Emphysema is a chronic disease that causes air to be trapped in the lungs; the alveoli become clogged with secretions or mucus and cannot expel the air. The person with emphysema appears pink in color. Breathing is assisted with the use of abdominal muscles; a barrel-type chest usually develops. The person with emphysema can be helped in expelling air by pursed-lip breathing. Pursed-lip breathing helps to slow the air expired, making it easier to breathe on inspiration.

The person with bronchitis, an inflammation of the bronchi, often has a bluish (cyanotic) appearance because of low levels of oxygen in the blood. Dyspnea, chronic cough, and production of much sputum are characteristic.

In general, the elderly person with chronic obstructive pulmonary disease has difficulty in expiring air; has an accumulation of air in the lungs; has some wheezing on breathing; and relies on accessory muscles, such as abdominal muscles, to breathe. These people may become quite anxious and apprehensive if an acute attack occurs. The geriatric nursing assistant should remain calm and summon the nurse in charge.

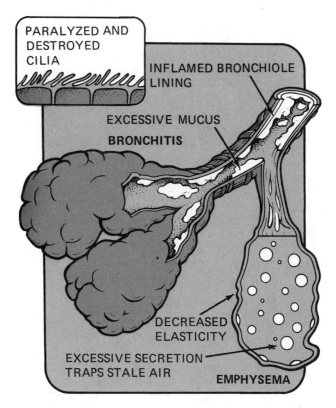

Figure 11.14. Chronic bronchitis and emphysema are obstructive pulmonary diseases.

TREATMENT

Treatment prescribed will include medications to help the dilation of bronchial and alveolar structures. The person will be asked to stop smoking. Oxygen therapy may be needed. Some people have an oxygen supply nearby so they can use it as necessary. Postural drainage, which requires that the person be in various positions in bed to allow the chest to drain of secretions, may be ordered. Antibiotics may also be ordered if the person's sputum indicates a sign of infection. Signs and symptoms of lung infections in persons with chronic obstructive pulmonary disease are:

> Increased cough; feeling of tightness in chest
> Increased sputum production
> Change in color of sputum from clear or white to yellow, green, or gray
> Change in consistency of sputum from thin and watery to thick, sticky, and stringy
> Increased shortness of breath and decreased exercise tolerance
> Fever and/or chills (temperature >100 °F, should notify charge nurse)
> Sudden decrease in the amount of sputum coughed up

Rehabilitation programs have been designed to help individuals with obstructive pulmonary disease to live as normal a life as possible. Breathing exercises, oxygen as needed, body exercise routines, and a healthy diet have been added to the treatment regime. The resident must learn to perform activity with a minimum of stress on the respiratory system. This means that maximum strength must be built into other muscles through a prescribed exercise program. Other devices, such as blow bottles and incentive spirometers, are used to help improve ventilation.

Geriatric Nursing Assistant Responses

1. Remain as calm as possible when assisting with care.
2. Report any sudden changes in condition that might indicate an acute attack or infection is beginning.
3. Assist resident with exercise routines as ordered.
4. Encourage a healthy diet. Make eating time as pleasant as possible.
5. Follow oxygen safety measures when oxygen is in use.
6. Encourage participation in social activities.
7. Provide for periods of rest.
8. Assist resident with postural drainage.
9. Assist resident to conserve energy and to use other body muscles to help do the work required.

KEY POINTS

1. Smoking is probably the leading irritant for people with chronic obstructive pulmonary disease.
2. Asthma is due to sensitivity to inhaled irritants.
3. Emphysema results from an inability to expel air easily. People with emphysema develop a barrel-type chest.

4. Bronchitis is a chronic inflammation of the bronchi. People with bronchitis have a bluish color to the skin.

5. The geriatric nursing assistant should remain calm in the care of people with COPD and be on the alert for signs and symptoms of an acute attack or infection of the lungs.

SELF-CHECK

1. Emphysema is characterized by _____ color of the skin and by a type of breathing, which is called _____ .

2. Name three irritants that can cause an asthmatic attack.

3. Chronic bronchitis is characterized by what three signs?

4. Mr. Callahan is 78 years old. He has been a heavy smoker for 40 years. He has great difficulty in performing simple care, such as brushing his teeth, because of his dyspnea and coughing spells. He is supposed to do his postural drainage each morning (Figure 11.15). List five nursing measures to assist him in his care and yet help him to be as independent as possible.

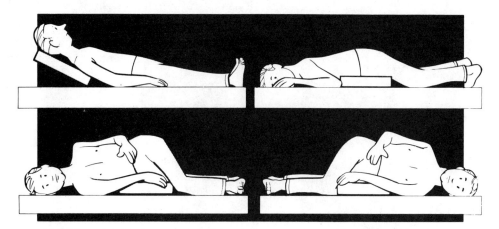

Figure 11.15. Upper left shows usual (non-postural) position. The remaining three positions show variations that are conducive to postural drainage. Positions will vary according to physician's orders.

SUGGESTED ACTIVITIES

1. Visit the Lung Association to learn of the activities there for people with COPD. Ask about the program for asthmatics and what is done to help smokers.

2. Talk with a respiratory therapist about the kinds of treatment available for COPD patients.

3. Visit a respiratory care department to learn how the equipment used in treatment is operated, and for what purposes.

CLINICAL APPLICATION

Using the problem-solving worksheet provided at the end of this unit, select a resident with chronic obstructive pulmonary disease and provide geriatric nursing assistant responses.

Cardiovascular Disease: Age-Related Changes

TERMINAL PERFORMANCE OBJECTIVE

Given information on the cardiovascular system and appropriate geriatric nursing assistant responses, be able to provide geriatric nursing assistant responses to residents with cardiovascular disease and to those who experience cardiac arrest.

Enabling Objectives

1. Identify five risk factors that predispose a person to heart disease.
2. Define atherosclerosis, angina, congestive heart failure (CHF), coronary occlusion, and myocardial infarction (MI).
3. Identify eight signs and symptoms of a possible heart attack.
4. Identify geriatric nursing assistant responses for residents with cardiovascular disease.
5. Review the procedures for cardiopulmonary resuscitation (CPR).
6. Apply geriatric nursing assistant responses to residents with cardiovascular diseases.

REVIEW SECTION

The topics the geriatric nursing assistant should review with the instructor are the age-related changes in the cardiovascular system, circulation of the blood through the heart and to the lungs and back, and cardiopulmonary resuscitation (CPR).

THE DISEASE AND ITS COURSE

Heart disease remains the leading cause of death in the United States; however, it is on the decrease because people are doing more to combat it. There are several risk factors which, if present, contribute to a person's likelihood of having a heart disease or heart attack. These factors are: obesity, smoking, hypertension, lack of exercise, heredity, too much cholesterol in the diet, and diabetes.

Atherosclerosis, referred to as hardening of the arteries, contributes to the majority of heart attacks in the United States. Atherosclerosis is the clogging of the inner lining of the arteries due to a major buildup of plaque or deposits of fat and calcium. Atherosclerosis can clog the coronary arteries and cause a coronary occlusion (Figure 11.16), or can clog the circulation to heart muscle and cause a myocardial infarction (MI). See figure 11.17a, b, and c.

Angina is pain in the vessels leading to the heart because of a decrease in the blood supply. This is usually brought on because of emotional or physical stress.

Congestive heart failure (CHF) is a state of the heart in which it is no longer able to pump an adequate supply of blood throughout the body. The resident will accumulate fluid throughout the body and be very dyspneic (short of breath).

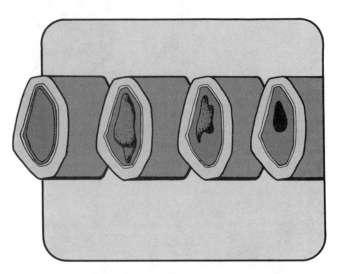

Figure 11.16. Atherosclerosis: The process of plaque formation.

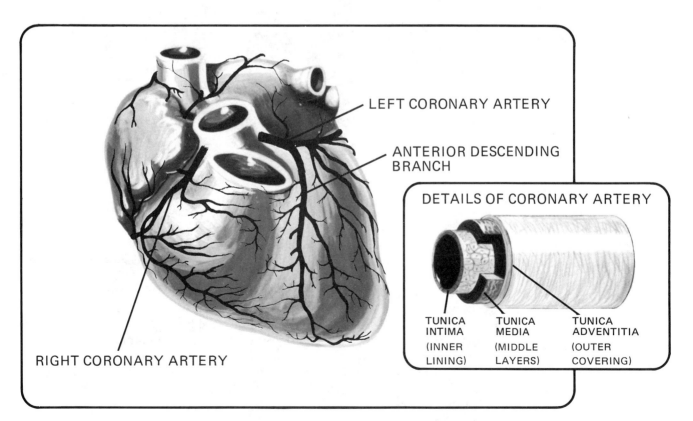

Figure 11.17(a). Normal heart.

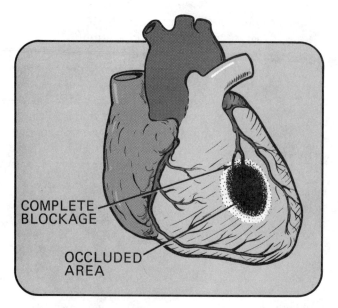

Figure 11.17(b).   Relationship of arterial disease and heart disease.

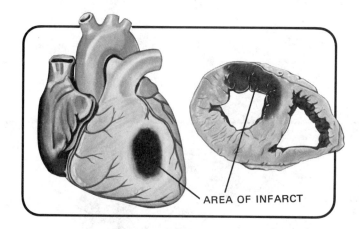

Figure 11.17(c).   Cross section of a myocardial infarction.

TREATMENT

It is important to know what the heart condition is that the resident has in order to provide adequate nursing responses. In general, there are some nursing responses to consider regardless of the heart disease. These responses include providing adequate rest for the person and some activity. Doctor's orders should reflect the amount of activity a resident can have. Diet becomes a key because it will regulate the amount of sodium (or salt) the resident may have and will place a limit on other foods in order to keep the person's weight at a desirable limit. Oxygen therapy may be ordered for periods of dyspnea. Positioning in bed is usually in a Fowler's or semi-Fowler's position. During peak times of acute respiratory distress, the 90-degree Fowler's or orthopneic position is ordered. This requires the person to be sitting straight up with pillows to support the back and a pillow on the overbed table, up close to the person so that he or she can rest his or her head.

Symptoms that should be reported immediately are acute difficulty in breathing, anxiety, apprehension, restlessness, weakness, perspiration, rapid pulse, dizziness, and chest pain. These may indicate a sudden change in the circulatory system or that a blood clot has entered a dangerous area.

Treatment of the person with heart disease is directed at reducing the work of the heart and at relief of pain when it occurs. Bedrest and activity must be balanced. Usually, a diet low in salt is ordered to help reduce fluid retention. Swelling of the lower extremities and fluid retention throughout the body may become a problem. The doctor will order medications (diuretics) to help rid the body of excess fluids. Medications (forms of digitalis) are ordered to improve the heart's tone and increase the strength of contractions. These medications help the heart to pump blood throughout the cardiovascular system. Oxygen therapy may also be needed when the resident is getting insufficient amounts. The person with an acute episode of illness will require hospitalization. Any sign of an acute attack needs to be reported immediately. Pain medication may be needed at this time. Many older people do not experience pain with a heart attack. The nursing assistant, therefore, must be alert to the other symptoms. If a cardiac arrest occurs, the care giver needs to know if the person is to receive cardiopulmonary resuscitation. Generally, each care giver in a health care institution is required to know how to administer cardiopulmonary resuscitation (CPR).

To provide CPR, the geriatric nursing assistant must be trained by a certified teacher and pass the written and practical tests. Satisfactory completion of a training program will qualify the completer with a CPR card. Figures 11.18 to 11.20 show the procedures for CPR. Reading these pages does not qualify the reader to perform CPR. Your instructor will assist you in becoming certified.

The American Red Cross and the American Heart Association offer courses of instruction in CPR. Every health care worker should complete one of these courses to be ready for emergency cardiac arrests.

Geriatric Nursing Assistant Responses

The following responses will help you to provide care to residents with cardiovascular disease.

1. Assist the resident with personal care, conserving energy and preventing fatigue.
2. Balance activities with rest periods as prescribed.
3. Monitor special diet and any salt restrictions.
4. Provide comfortable positions for residents whether they are in bed or in a wheelchair. Breathing is easier when the body is upright and supported.
5. Monitor swelling of the lower extremities. Elevate feet, if authorized. (This might not be desirable at all times.)
6. Watch for any sudden change, such as dyspnea, anxiety, and chest pain, and report immediately. Do not rely on pain to occur.
7. Follow the procedures for oxygen safety.
8. Monitor intake and output. Resident may be on diuretics to monitor fluid loss.
9. Monitor weight as ordered. Weight will indicate body fluid loss (see response 8).
10. Be prepared to do CPR. Become certified through the Red Cross or Heart Association.

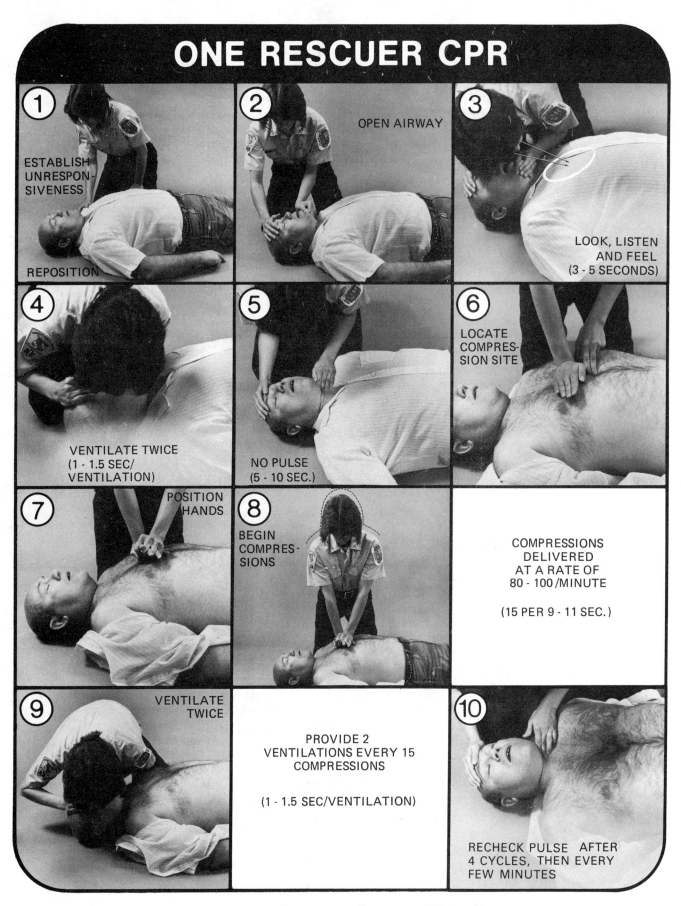

Figure 11.18. One-rescuer CPR.

TWO RESCUER CPR

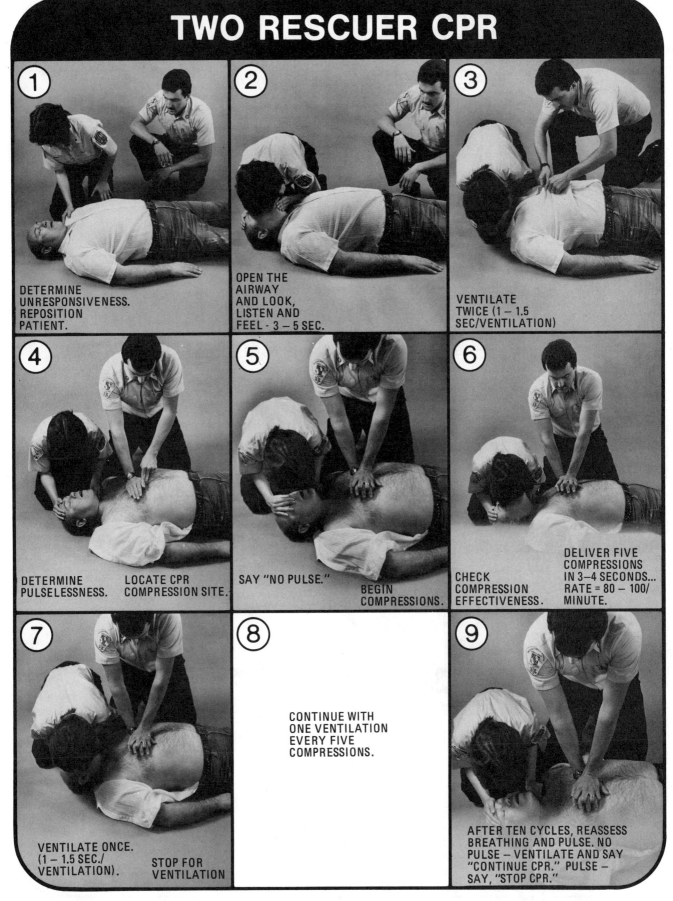

1 DETERMINE UNRESPONSIVENESS. REPOSITION PATIENT.

2 OPEN THE AIRWAY AND LOOK, LISTEN AND FEEL - 3 — 5 SEC.

3 VENTILATE TWICE (1 — 1.5 SEC/VENTILATION)

4 DETERMINE PULSELESSNESS.   LOCATE CPR COMPRESSION SITE.

5 SAY "NO PULSE."   BEGIN COMPRESSIONS.

6 CHECK COMPRESSION EFFECTIVENESS.   DELIVER FIVE COMPRESSIONS IN 3–4 SECONDS... RATE = 80 — 100/ MINUTE.

7 VENTILATE ONCE. (1 — 1.5 SEC./ VENTILATION).   STOP FOR VENTILATION

8 CONTINUE WITH ONE VENTILATION EVERY FIVE COMPRESSIONS.

9 AFTER TEN CYCLES, REASSESS BREATHING AND PULSE. NO PULSE — VENTILATE AND SAY "CONTINUE CPR." PULSE — SAY, "STOP CPR."

Figure 11.19.   Two-rescuer CPR.

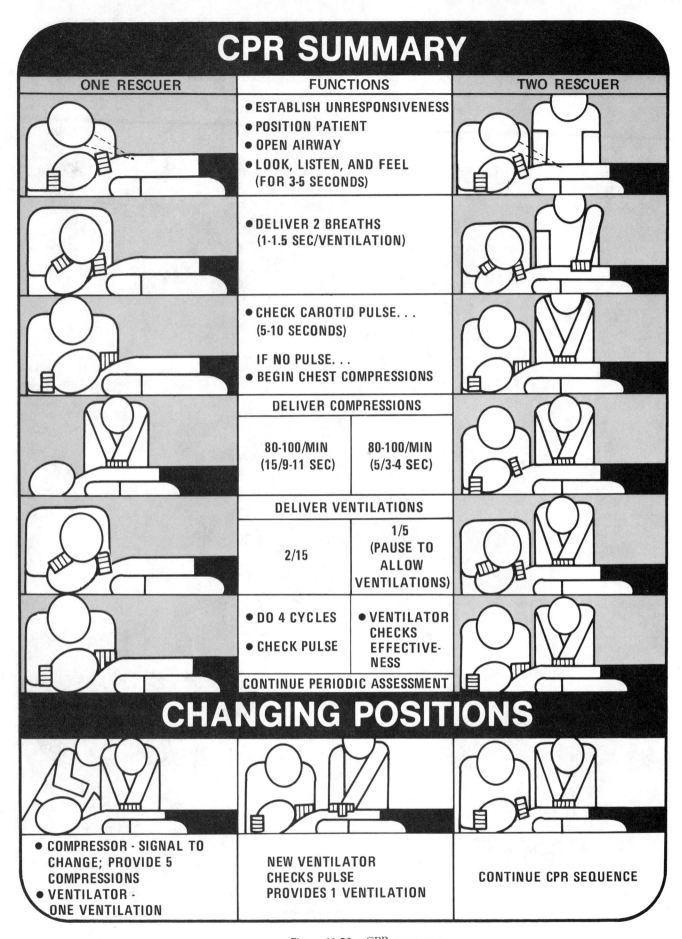

Figure 11.20.   CPR summary.

KEY POINTS

1. There are at least seven risk factors that predispose people to heart disease, the leading cause of death of the elderly.
2. Atherosclerosis becomes worse with aging and is an underlying factor in cardiovascular diseases.
3. The geriatric nursing assistant should be alert to the eight signs of an impending heart attack.
4. Geriatric nursing assistant responses include preparation in CPR. Every geriatric nursing assistant should take the course taught by a certified CPR teacher and receive a card of CPR certification.

SELF-CHECK

1. Identify five risk factors for heart disease.

2. Define the following terms.
   a. Hypertension

   b. Angina

   c. Myocardial infarction

   d. Coronary occlusion

   e. Congestive heart failure

3. State eight signs and symptoms of an impending heart attack.

4. Identify five geriatric nursing assistant responses for people with cardiovascular disease.

5. When doing CPR, what is the number of compressions per minute for an adult?

6. When one person is doing CPR, how many breaths to how many compressions are given?

7. When a pulse is felt after giving a series of compressions and breaths, do you continue CPR or stop? Why?

8. Describe the position of the hands for compressions when doing CPR.

SUGGESTED ACTIVITIES

1. Complete a course in CPR and earn your card that certifies you.
2. Visit the American Red Cross and learn about their activities of instruction in CPR.
3. Visit the American Heart Association to learn about the activities they do in trying to prevent heart disease.
4. Talk with a family member or friend who had a heart attack. Find out what it was like for that person.

CLINICAL APPLICATION

Using the problem-solving worksheet provided at the end of this unit, select a resident with cardiovascular disease and provide geriatric nursing assistant responses.

WORKSHEET

Implications for Care of an Elderly Cognitively Impaired Person with Alzheimer's Disease or Related Disorder and Family Members

Directions: Select an elderly, cognitively impaired person and outline implications for care for the person and for family members.

Description of the elderly person: (First name; age and sex; diagnosis; family/social history; former occupation; present living situation; strengths and weaknesses in functioning and ability to do activities of daily living.)

Needs/problems: (Review body systems and make a list of specific problem areas.)

Outline care needed: (Based on problems identified.)

Describe family members: (List each person by relationship—husband, son, daughter, and so on, and identify role changes and emotional, social, and physical problems, if any.)

List family support systems: (Identify what resources family uses to help with caring for the cognitively impaired person.)

List any additional implications for care that can be identified and how this care can be provided: (i.e., use of respite care givers or adult care center to relieve family care giver).

WORKSHEET

Nursing Responses: Cerebral Vascular Accident

Directions: Select a resident and apply geriatric nursing assistant responses. Evaluate for progress toward independent living.

Resident: _____   *Diagnosis:* _____
     (initials only)

Description of the resident: (Briefly describe the person: age, sex, physical and emotional characteristics)

Nursing assistant responses:
Needs   Nursing Responses

Physical:

Emotional:

Progress toward
independent living:

WORKSHEET

Nursing Responses: Diabetes Mellitus

Directions: Select a resident and apply geriatric nursing assistant responses. Evaluate for progress toward independent living.

Resident: _____   *Diagnosis:* _____
       (initials only)

Description of the resident: (Briefly describe the person: age, sex, physical and emotional characteristics)

Nursing assistant responses:
Needs   Nursing Responses
Physical:

Emotional:

Progress toward
independent living:

WORKSHEET

Nursing Responses: Cancer

Directions: Select a resident and apply geriatric nursing assistant responses. Evaluate for progress toward independent living.

Resident: _____   *Diagnosis:* _____
         (initials only)

Description of the resident: (Briefly describe the person: age, sex, physical and emotional characteristics)

Nursing assistant responses:
Needs   Nursing Responses
Physical:

Emotional:

Progress toward
independent living:

WORKSHEET

Nursing Responses: Arthritis

Directions: Select a resident and apply geriatric nursing assistant responses. Evaluate for progress toward independent living.

Resident: _____   *Diagnosis:* _____
           (initials only)

Description of the resident: (Briefly describe the person: age, sex, physical and emotional characteristics)

Nursing assistant responses:

Needs   Nursing Responses

Physical:

Emotional:

Progress toward
independent living:

WORKSHEET

Nursing Responses: Obstructive Pulmonary Disease

Directions: Select a resident and apply geriatric nursing assistant responses.
Evaluate for progress toward independent living.

Resident: _____   *Diagnosis:* _____
          (initials only)

Description of the resident: (Briefly describe the person: age, sex, physical
and emotional characteristics)

Nursing assistant responses:
Needs   Nursing Responses
Physical:

Emotional:

Progress toward
independent living:

WORKSHEET

Nursing Responses: Cardiovascular Disease

Directions: Select a resident and apply geriatric nursing assistant responses. Evaluate for progress toward independent living.

Resident: _____   *Diagnosis:* _____
        (initials only)

Description of the resident: (Briefly describe the person: age, sex, physical and emotional characteristics)

Nursing assistant responses:

Needs   **Nursing Responses**

Physical:

Emotional:

Progress toward
independent living:

12 GRIEVING, DYING, AND DEATH

TERMINAL PERFORMANCE OBJECTIVE

Given information on the processes involved with grieving, dying, and death and the needs of the care giver in these situations, be able to apply appropriate geriatric nursing assistant responses to residents who are dying and to other family members while maintaining care of one's own needs.

Enabling Objectives

1. Describe the stages of grieving and dying proposed by Elizabeth Kübler-Ross.
2. Self-examine feelings as a care giver about dying and death.
3. Identify coping techniques as a care giver.
4. Describe the concept of hospice care.
5. Identify general nursing assistant procedures for residents who die.
6. Apply geriatric nursing assistant responses to a dying resident and his or her family members.

REVIEW SECTION

The topics the geriatric nursing assistant should review with the instructor are communication techniques and postmortem care.

THE GRIEVING RESIDENT AND FAMILY MEMBERS

The person who is dying grieves for his or her loss of life and experiences certain stages which have been described by Elizabeth Kübler-Ross, a psychiatrist who has been working with dying people for many years. She has described five stages experienced by dying people (Figure 12.1). Loved ones who observe a family member dying also experience similar stages.

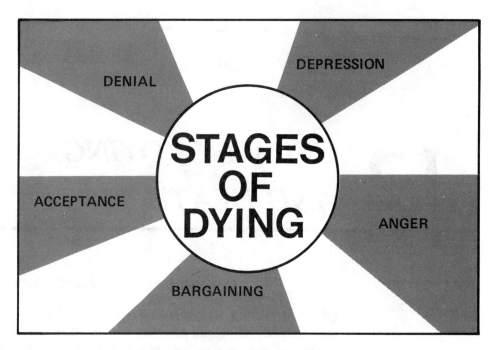

Figure 12.1.

These stages are (Figure 12.2):

Denial.	The person speaks of an incorrect diagnosis or refuses to believe that death will come. Family members will also deny the possibility of death.
Anger.	The dying person may say, "Why did this have to happen to me?" The person may demonstrate anger with irritable expressions, may lash out at workers or family members. Family members may blame doctors, nurses, or another person.
Bargaining.	The dying person realizes that death will occur but may want to live until a certain event occurs. Family members may hope the person will live until "all family members arrive."
Depression.	The dying person becomes sad about losing his or her life and leaving family and dear ones. He or she accepts that death will occur. Family members may express their sadness through tears and very quiet behavior.
Acceptance.	The dying person may show a calmness and prepares to finish "unfinished" business. He or she may give away favorite belongings. Family assist in the process. They try to keep the person free of any worry or anxiety about unfinished business.

Figure 12.2.   The stages of grieving and dying.

The stages of grieving and dying usually fluctuate. In some instances, the dying person may stay in one stage and never seem to move to acceptance even when death is about to occur. Family members may refuse to admit that their loved one will die. The geriatric nursing assistant must try to understand what the grieving person and family members are experiencing. Sometimes just being there to listen to the dying person and family members helps (Figure 12.3). It is wrong to give false hope and say that "it will be all right" when you and they know that is not the case. Sometimes involving the family members in part of the care helps them to feel useful and contributing.

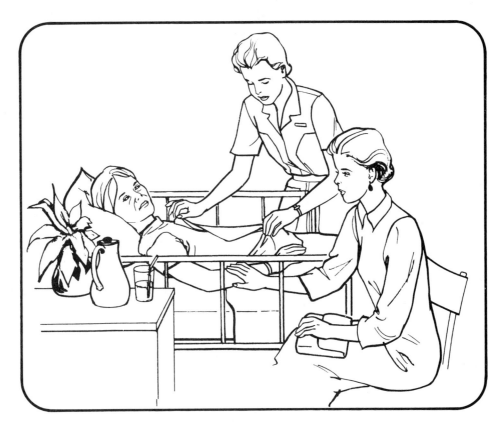

Figure 12.3.

Self-Care for the Care Givers

It is essential that as a care giver, the geriatric nursing assistant examines his or her own feelings and values about death. To be helpful to other people who are dying, the geriatric nursing assistant must have a strong sense of what death means, must be able to accept it, and must be able to provide appropriate responses to dying people and family members. A worksheet has been provided to help you think through feelings about death. Empathy and effective communication skills are very valuable at this time. The geriatric nursing assistant should not try swaying the dying person and family members to agree with his or her beliefs but must be supportive and accepting of the beliefs held by the dying person and family.

A social worker, psychologist, member of the clergy, or a trained professional can be excellent resources when a resident is dying. These professionals are trained to work with grieving families and can help them to work through

WORKSHEET: PERSONAL FEELINGS REGARDING DEATH AND DYING

Directions: Consider the following statements and write your feelings about death and dying.

1. My first experience with death in my life was:

2. My first experience with a dying resident was:

3. I think death is:

4. My closest relative to die was: _____ . I felt:

5. My family looks upon death as:

6. When a member of my family is very ill and may die, we always: (Describe the rituals or usual activities your family does.)

7. If I were told I had a fatal illness, I would want to do the following:

8. When I care for a dying resident, I feel like:

9. When I care for a resident who has died, I feel like:

10. Add anything else you feel about dying and death.

the grieving process. These same professionals can assist the geriatric nursing assistant sort through mixed emotions and feelings during these times. Care givers must have an opportunity to discuss pent-up emotions and find a way to "fill their cups" with the ability to go on caring. Many care givers become very fond and grow to love residents they have known for weeks, months, and years. "Care givers conferences" routinely established to provide for talking-out emotions can be a great support mechanism and help to relieve stress caused by the emotions. In addition, the geriatric nursing assistant should try to follow the guidelines below, which may help in coping:

1. Plan a reward for yourself, no matter how small, to help replenish some of the emotion you give away. Do something that is fun, enjoyable.
2. Establish friendships away from the job so that you can ventilate feelings that become "pent up." Have someone you can talk to about feelings, with whom you can cry and feel okay about it. (Be sure to maintain confidentiality about clients, if discussed.)
3. If you have nagging thoughts about something you should have done and have not, plan a time and do it. Nagging thoughts make you feel guilty and less free and add more stress than you need.

Nursing Responses to Grieving Residents and Family Members

1. Spend as much time as possible with the resident; let family members know that you are available.
2. Give attention to the resident in view of family members; maintain empathy and tact; attend to family needs.
3. Maintain an appropriate approach; respond to the needs of the resident as they change.
4. Render all responses with respect and dignity for the person and family.
5. Administer to resident as though he or she will live; do not ignore requests as though they are meaningless.
6. Respect all resident's rights.
7. Allow resident to make choices and decisions about care.
8. Report need for pain medication immediately.
9. Seek and honor religious preferences.
10. Keep the resident as comfortable as possible.

Nursing Assistant Responses for the Dying Resident

The person who is dying has some physical changes that require frequent attention. Usually, the person perspires profusely. The bed linens need changing to keep the person dry (Figure 12.4). The mouth drops open and mouth breathing produces dryness and coating of the tongue. Lips might become quite dry. Mouth care is needed frequently. The skin may appear mottled (bluish discoloration in patches over the skin, especially in the lower extremities). Edema (fluid in the tissues) and mottling require frequent position changes. The skin may feel cool. Respiration slows considerably and may become erratic (Cheyne-Stokes respiration). The pulse becomes weak, thready, and barely palpable.

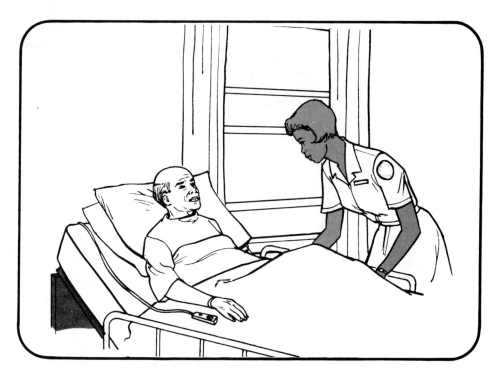

Figure 12.4.

Although the dying person's vision may not be intact, hearing may still be acute. Care givers and family members should not say anything they do not want the dying person to hear. Whispering should be avoided. Speak to the dying person with a moderate tone you ordinarily would use, and apply touch with caring and concern. Respect and dignity for the dying person at all times should be the guiding principle.

CHECKLIST FOR CARE OF THE DYING RESIDENT

	Yes	*No*
1. Provide frequent attention to emotional concerns (loneliness, fear, etc.) of resident and family.	—	—
2. Provide for spiritual concerns (preferred member of the clergy is called).	—	—
3. Maintain privacy.	—	—
4. Monitor vital signs frequently or as ordered.	—	—
5. Provide personal care, and comfort; bathe and change linens as necessary.	—	—
6. Maintain resident in Fowler's position or head elevated as needed.	—	—
7. Observe for mucus accumulation in the mouth; report need for suctioning.	—	—
8. Provide oral hygiene frequently.	—	—
9. Change position at least every 2 hours.	—	—
10. Provide perineal care as necessary.	—	—

	Yes	No
11. Provide liquids as tolerated, and monitor intake and output.	—	—
12. Keep room ventilated and cheerful.	—	—
13. Keep environment uncluttered.	—	—
14. Keep bedrails up at all times.	—	—
15. Monitor oxygen supply and report when low.	—	—
16. Provide for oxygen safety.	—	—

HOSPICE PROGRAMS

The word *hospice* has become synonymous with care of the terminally ill. The word itself means a resting place. The program of care that is known as hospice provides care for the patient and help for the family. If the dying person is at home, the home becomes the primary center of care, which is provided by family members or friends who are taught basic nursing. The focus of care is on pain control and death with dignity. Family members are provided ongoing emotional support through a team of care givers who are interdisciplinary; care is provided 7 days a week, 24 hours a day.

The hospice program provides for continued education and training of all its staff members in order to meet the needs of the terminally ill residents and family members. A nursing assistant working in a hospice program is a vital member of the care-giving team. Hospice programs involve volunteers to supplement care services. The family is the center of the hospice team.

The hospice concept has become an integral part of most health care institutions, including hospitals, nursing homes, and home health agencies. In hospitals and nursing homes there may be a pastoral care team made up of religious workers, nurses, and social workers who counsel the clients and family members, helping them to work through their grief. Special meetings might be held to help family members discuss their feelings and to work through a plan that will help them to organize their days after the person expires. A special feature of the hospice program is continued support for family members after the terminally ill person expires.

CARE OF THE PERSON WHO DIES

The geriatric nursing assistant who prepares the deceased person should continue to honor the body with dignity and respect.

If the family wants to see the body for the last time, do the following:

1. Flatten the bed and straighten the body.
2. Cover the body, bringing the bed linens up to the chin. Arrange the bed linens neatly.
3. Close the eyes (Figure 12.5).
4. Prop up the chin with a rolled towel to support closure of the mouth. (Pull bed linens over the towel.)
5. Arrange room neatly.
6. Provide privacy for the family.

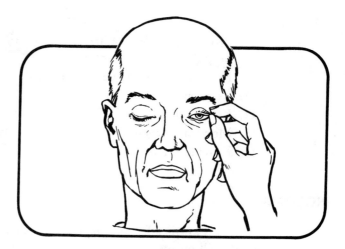

Figure 12.5.

Each facility will have its own policies for care of the body. Postmortem care has changed drastically through the years. (In the past, the anal opening had to be packed and the body was tied at the wrists and ankles.) Morticians from funeral parlors do not expect extensive postmortem care any more. The general geriatric nursing assistant responses should include the following:

1. The body is thoroughly cleansed (Figure 12.6). Keep the body covered and provide privacy as usual.
2. All dressings are changed and replaced with clean ones. Tubes are removed.
3. The hair should be combed.
4. Dentures may or may not be replaced. Check with the funeral parlor.
5. The body is placed in alignment, arms and legs straightened.
6. Surrounding doors are usually closed when the body is removed by the funeral parlor.
7. Belongings are gathered and given to family members. All valuables should be given to a family member. (Notations need to be entered on the resident's record. Be sure to check with the nurse in charge regarding what valuables and belongings are given to family members.)

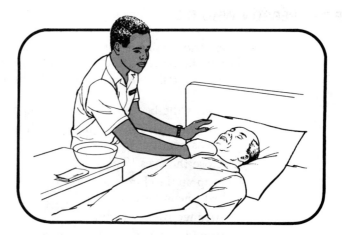

Figure 12.6.

Family members also need attention. The geriatric nursing assistant should be available to them and respond to questions and concerns. Be there to listen and to show caring about their loss. Participate, if possible, in services for the deceased if these are part of the activities provided by the facility. Family members will appreciate the attendance of staff members at these ceremonies.

KEY POINTS

1. A dying resident should have needs met: physical, social, psychological, and spiritual, as he/she experiences the emotional stages of dying.
2. Spiritual needs may gain in significance for dying residents.
3. Family members may have a need to express their grief; they may experience stages similar to the grief process of the dying person. The hospice concept and program can be very meaningful to the dying person, and especially to grieving family members.
4. Hospice programs should have a goal of continuing support to family members *after* the resident passes on.
5. The geriatric nursing assistant has a contributing role in the care of dying residents, in meeting the emotional needs of family members, and in care of the resident after death.
6. The geriatric nursing assistant must find ways to cope with loss of residents and to "refill the cup" enabling him or her to care.

SELF-CHECK

1. List the psychological stages of grief and dying that have been described by Elizabeth Kübler-Ross, the reknowned psychiatrist.

2. When a resident expresses the wish to live until "my daughter gets married," this is the stage of _____ .
3. The expression "The doctor is wrong; this cannot happen to me" is the stage of _____ .
4. When the resident withdraws and cries, showing much sadness over the terminal diagnosis, the stage of _____ has occurred.
5. The _____ stage has occurred when the resident wants to make arrangements for belongings and asks to have a will made.

True or False. Place a T in front of statements that are true, and F in front of statements that are false.

_____ 6. All stages are experienced by all grieving people.
_____ 7. A grieving person may fluctuate back and forth from one stage to another.
_____ 8. The nursing assistant's contribution to grieving family members may be mainly one of listening.

_____ 9. The nursing assistant can be more help to grieving residents if he/she understands personal feelings about dying and death.

_____ 10. Most dying residents want to be left alone.

_____ 11. Care of the deceased resident is conducted as though he/she were still living.

_____ 12. Hospice programs center on total care of the client.

SUGGESTED ACTIVITIES

1. Visit with a social worker or pastoral care worker to learn of reactions family members have had to the dying and death of a loved one.
2. Attend a support group session that deals with the hospice concept.
3. Inquire at a hospital and a nursing home about how hospice programs are organized.
4. Complete the worksheet on examining your feelings about dying and death. Discuss with your classmates.

CLINICAL APPLICATION

Using the guidelines and checklist in this unit, select a resident who is terminally ill or close to death. Apply the suggested nursing responses and write a report about the care given, your feelings about caring for the resident, and the resident's reactions. Add anything else you would like to describe or explain. If family members were involved, include their reactions.

13 SPECIAL CARE SERIES

TERMINAL PERFORMANCE OBJECTIVE

Given information about residents with special forms of treatment and appropriate geriatric nursing assistant responses, be able to provide these responses when caring for residents with these special treatments.

Enabling Objectives

1. Describe a tracheostomy, and state why it is needed.
2. Identify five geriatric nursing assistant responses for a person with a tracheostomy.
3. Describe the purpose of oxygen therapy.
4. Identify five geriatric nursing assistant responses to maintaining oxygen safety.
5. Identify five geriatric nursing assistant responses for residents receiving oxygen therapy.
6. Describe the purpose of casts.
7. Identify five geriatric nursing assistant responses for resident with casts.
8. Describe the purpose of traction.
9. Identify five geriatric nursing assistant responses for residents with traction.
10. Identify three reasons why geriatric nursing assistants must be aware of possible drug reactions.
11. Identify five common drug reactions that need to be reported immediately.
12. Apply appropriate geriatric nursing assistant responses to residents with these special treatments.

REVIEW SECTION

The topics the geriatric nursing assistant should review with the instructor are the anatomy and physiology of the respiratory system, oxygen therapy, types of casts, and types of traction.

NURSING ASSISTANT RESPONSES FOR RESIDENTS WITH TRACHEOSTOMIES

A tracheostomy is a surgical procedure that involves making an opening into the trachea. It is an opening that is maintained by the insertion of a tracheostomy tube, which can be made of plastic, silver, or nylon. The purpose of the tracheostomy is to establish and maintain an airway so that the person can breathe. A tracheostomy is necessary when some obstruction has occurred to prevent the person from gaining oxygen any other way, such as severe burns to the respiratory tract, tumors, or paralysis of the vocal cords.

The tube has holes on each side of the opening through which cloth tapes are inserted. These tapes then tie around the person's neck to keep the tube from being coughed out of position. If the tube is coughed out, the opening may close and cut off the person's air supply.

Although care of the tracheostomy tube is not a nursing assistant function, it is necessary for the nursing assistant to understand what to expect and what to report if problems should occur. The person who must have a tracheostomy might be quite fearful and apprehensive since he or she will not be able to talk. A communication system must be established and emotional support provided to help the person relax. Review and study the checklist, which will help you understand what to report to your supervisor.

CHECKLIST FOR CARE OF A RESIDENT WITH A TRACHEOSTOMY TUBE (Figure 13.1)

	Yes	No
1. Provide for the appropriate licensed person to suction resident when airway becomes plugged, breathing is noisy, respirations are increased, and pulse rate increased. Suction machine should be in good working order at the bedside.	—	—
2. Provide care for resident in calm, relaxed manner.	—	—
3. Check skin around tracheostomy for irritation. Report irritation to licensed nurse.	—	—
4. Provide Fowler's or modified position according to orders and resident's comfort.	—	—
5. Check to see if safety hemostat or tracheal dilator is at bedside (used in case tube is coughed up).	—	—
6. Establish a communication system. It must be understood and used by all staff.	—	—
7. Place call signal within resident's reach at all times.	—	—
8. Apply oxygen safety precautions if oxygen is in use.	—	—
9. Check humidifier for proper operation when in use.	—	—

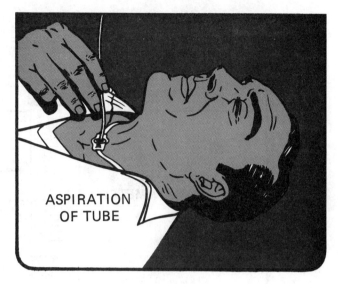

ASPIRATION
OF TUBE

Figure 13.1.

	Yes	No
10. Monitor nutrition, intake and output. (Nutritional state may be difficult to maintain.)	—	—
11. Provide for diversional activities as tolerated.	—	—

KEY POINTS

1. Residents with tracheostomies need careful observation for respiratory obstruction. Know the signs/symptoms.
2. Insertion of a tracheostomy tube is a sterile procedure and not in the caregiving realm of the nursing assistant. Report when care of the tube needs to be done.
3. Observe and report any unusual reactions of resident immediately.

NURSING ASSISTANT RESPONSES FOR RESIDENTS RECEIVING OXYGEN

Oxygen therapy is provided to clients who have difficulty in breathing a sufficient amount. The doctor prescribes oxygen and determines how much should be given. The licensed nurse sets the amount of oxygen by adjusting the gauge on the equipment, which is attached to the source of oxygen (Figure 13.2).

In hospitals the supply of oxygen comes from a wall unit that is hooked to a central supply. Many nursing homes still use the large tanks of oxygen which are transported from a storage area on a special cart to the resident's bedside.

The resident receives oxygen by using a mask or a nasal cannula. See figure 13.3a and b. Either of these pieces of equipment are attached by tube to the source of oxygen. The oxygen passes from the source, through water, to the resident. It is necessary to moisten the oxygen because otherwise the dryness of the oxygen would cause irritation to the mucous membranes. The supply of water must be maintained as well as the supply of oxygen. There is a portable tank of oxygen which can be attached to a wheelchair. These tanks do not last very long and must be checked frequently to assure a supply.

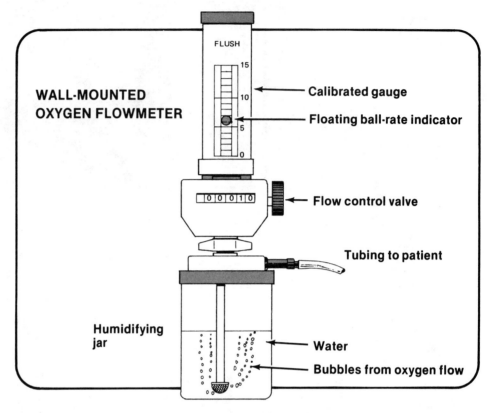

FLUSH

WALL-MOUNTED
OXYGEN FLOWMETER

15

10

5

0

00010

←—— Calibrated gauge

←—— Floating ball-rate indicator

←—— Flow control valve

Tubing to patient

Humidifying
jar

←—— Water

←—— Bubbles from oxygen flow

Figure 13.2.

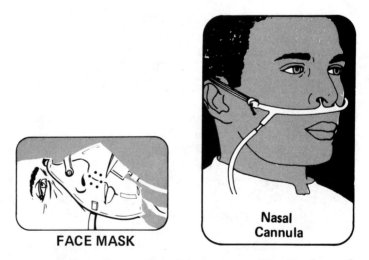

FACE MASK

Nasal
Cannula

Figure 13.3(a). Face mask.   Figure 13.3(b). Nasal cannula.

The resident who requires additional oxygen may become apprehensive easily. The inability to breathe sufficient quantities of air is conducive to this apprehensiveness. Residents may become fearful they will not be able to breathe at all.

Oxygen safety precautions must be observed at all times (Figure 13.4). Oxygen in a room that has a heat source and combustible materials may produce the perfect environment for a fire. Therefore, the standard oxygen safety rules must be followed. These rules are the following:

1. Do not use other electrical appliances when oxygen is being administered.
2. Post "no smoking" signs on door and in view of people entering room.
3. Avoid use of woolen blankets. (May cause a spark.)
4. Avoid using oil-based ointments (burnable).
5. Be sure oxygen tank is secured by a chain on a balanced cart when in use.
6. Be sure oxygen tank is chained on cart and gauge is closed when transporting tank.

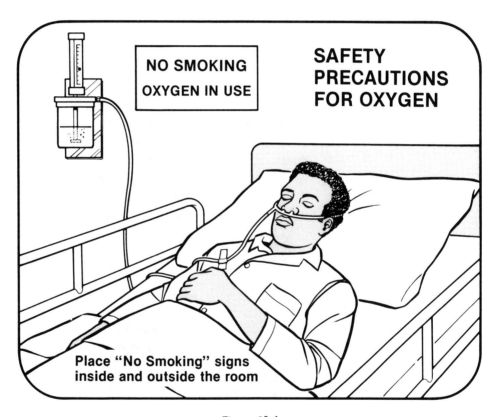

NO SMOKING

OXYGEN IN USE

SAFETY PRECAUTIONS FOR OXYGEN

Place "No Smoking" signs inside and outside the room

Figure 13.4.

A checklist has been included in this unit to help the geriatric nursing assistant provide for the comfort and safety of a person receiving oxygen.

CHECKLIST FOR RESIDENT RECEIVING OXYGEN

	Yes	*No*
1. Observe resident's emotional reaction to therapy.	—	—
2. Provide confidence and reassurance in nursing approach; remain calm.	—	—

	Yes	*No*
3. Provide for proper positioning—usually, modified Fowler's position.	—	—
4. Maintain cleanliness of mask and cannula. (Be sure the nares of cannula are kept clean.)	—	—
5. Monitor oxygen flow for:		
a. Humidity–water level (sterile water)	—	—
b. Liters of oxygen as ordered	—	—
c. Reserve oxygen in tank	—	—
d. Tank is secured on a cart with chain guard	—	—
6. Follow oxygen safety precautions.	—	—
7. Provide frequent mouth care—avoid oil-based ointments.	—	—
8. Maintain cleanliness and comfort of resident.	—	—
9. Observe and report untoward symptoms: dyspnea, cyanosis, restlessness, apprehension, tachypnea (rapid breathing).	—	—

KEY POINTS

1. Oxygen safety is the business of all personnel, especially the nursing assistant, who provides the most frequent care.
2. Know all safety measures and follow them.
3. Observe and report problems immediately.
4. Provide the geriatric nursing assistant responses when caring for resident receiving oxygen therapy.
5. Be able to operate a fire extinguisher.

NURSING ASSISTANT RESPONSES FOR RESIDENTS WITH CASTS

The purpose of a cast is immobilization of a body part to give it rest and time to heal. A cast is a type of bandage made from material coated with plaster of paris. When wet, it becomes very pliable and can be applied to most body parts. As the bandage dries, it becomes hard and serves to immobilize the part. Elderly residents are prone to fractures and may find themselves in a cast. Common fracture areas include the femur, the neck of the femur (commonly called hip fracture), and the wrist.

Before the cast is applied, bony surfaces are protected with padding and stockinette. Once the wet plaster of paris is in place, careful handling is required to make sure that no indentations form in the cast. Indentations can cause pressure areas and may result in a pressure sore developing which is not visible to the eye. Dryness and itching under the cast may prompt the resident to try to poke an object under the cast in order to scratch. This should not be allowed since a break in the skin might occur and that could lead to an unseen skin infection.

Fiberglass material is being used more frequently for making casts. Fiberglass casts are more advantageous because they dry quickly and are lighter in weight. The indentations of plaster of paris casts are avoided and the person does not become as tired when manipulating a lighter cast.

The checklist provided lists the geriatric nursing assistant responses for residents with casts. See also Figure 13.5.

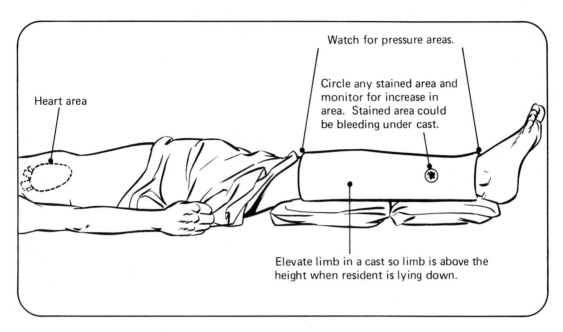

Figure 13.5. Elevate limb in cast so the limb is above the heart when resident is lying down. Circle any stained area and monitor for excessive bleeding in area.

CHECKLIST FOR CARE OF A RESIDENT WITH A CAST

When Cast Is Wet

	Yes	No
1. Touch the cast as little as possible and only with the palms of the hand, not the fingers.	—	—
2. Elevate the casted limb on several plastic-covered pillows (follow orders) for reduction of swelling that occurs in a recently injured limb. (Limb should be above level of the heart when resident is lying down.)	—	—
3. Turn resident at least every 2 hours to allow cast to dry evenly on all sides. Have help in the move.	—	—
4. Have resident assist if arms are free and bed is equipped with a trapeze. Resident can help lift body with use of the trapeze.	—	—
5. Keep resident covered but limb exposed to the air.	—	—
6. Provide privacy, as needed, of body parts that might be exposed.	—	—
7. Offer emotional support and reassurance as needed.	—	—
8. Check for pain and report immediately.	—	—
9. Observe extremities for any change if resident has arm or leg cast. Observe skin for color, temperature, tingling sensation or complaints of numbness, and lack of movement of toes or fingers—whatever is appropriate.	—	—

	Yes	*No*
10. Observe for any color changes in cast if there is an area where bleeding might occur; circle area on cast with marker and report immediately.	—	—

When Cast Is Dry

	Yes	*No*
1. Continue to monitor for color changes in cast; for temperature and color of extremity; for complaints of numbness, tingling, or pain.	—	—
2. Check for pressure areas and burning sensation under the cast.	—	—
3. Monitor odors coming from cast—foul odor may mean infection.	—	—
4. Keep skin clean and lubricated.	—	—
5. Prevent edges of the cast from irritating skin.	—	—
6. Maintain body alignment.	—	—
7. Protect perineal areas of body casts by covering with plastic and changing plastic often.	—	—

KEY POINTS

1. Casts hide infections or problems that develop. Know the signs and symptoms of pressure, and infections, and report immediately.
2. Wet casts require careful handling.
3. Follow all nursing measures of immobile residents to help prevent complications of body systems.

NURSING ASSISTANT RESPONSES FOR RESIDENTS IN TRACTION

Traction is another way to immobilize a body part in order to place the part in alignment and to give it rest in order to allow time to heal. Traction involves two forces or pulls (Figure 13.6). One force or pull occurs through the use of

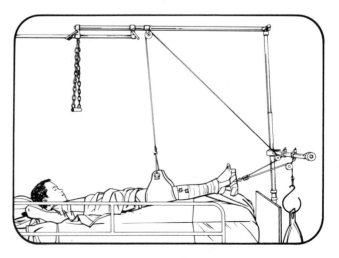

Figure 13.6.

weights and pulleys that are attached to the limb, as in the case of a broken arm or leg. The other force is the resident's body, serving to counteract the pull from the attached weights. Since the person is confined to bed, the nursing challenge is to prevent complications of immobility. The elderly person has a more difficult time in preventing complications because of the general decrease in body function before any additional reason for immobility occurs.

There are a number of different kinds of traction, depending on the body part to be immobilized. There is skin traction, which involves applying tape to the skin and attaching pulleys to the tape. There is also skeletal traction, in which wires or pins are placed directly into the bone and the weights and pulleys are attached to the pins or wires. Regardless of the type of traction, precautions to prevent complications and measures to help the resident keep comfortable are based on the same nursing principles.

Immobility of elderly people leads to many complications; therefore, consideration must be given to all body systems and measures provided to maintain and promote optimal functioning. The checklist for geriatric nursing assistants will help to prevent complications.

CHECKLIST FOR CARE OF A RESIDENT IN TRACTION

	Yes	No
1. Provide for resident's comfort; assess pain and report.	—	—
2. Check weights and pulleys for correct weight in place.	—	—
3. Check the ropes for freedom from obstruction. Weights should hang free without touching bedclothes, bed, and so on; no kinks or knots in ropes.	—	—
4. Line of traction is straight, resident's limb is in alignment with remainder of body.	—	—
5. Check resident's skin for pressure areas:		
a. Where traction is applied	—	—
b. Over bony surfaces: elbows, heels, sacrum, shoulders, and so on	—	—
6. Apply protective lotions to bony surfaces and massage areas well.	—	—
7. Maintain level position; head flat, unless ordered differently.	—	—
8. Check orders for exercises to maintain strength in unaffected limbs, in deep breathing, in coughing, and have resident do as ordered.	—	—
9. Monitor diet and eliminations—avoid constipation.	—	—
10. Encourage liquids, monitor I&O.	—	—
11. Provide diversional activities, prevent boredom.	—	—

KEY POINTS

1. Monitoring the resident in traction for any problems with equipment or alignment will prevent complications.
2. Immobile residents need nursing measures for all body systems in order to avoid complications.
3. Maintenance of as many body functions as possible will aid recovery.

4. The resident in traction needs diversional activities to help with the emotional and psychological effects of immobilization.

NURSING ASSISTANT RESPONSES FOR RESIDENTS WITH POSSIBLE DRUG REACTION

The geriatric nursing assistant can play a major role in care of the elderly by being aware of possible side effects of drugs elderly residents receive. The aging person is vulnerable to side effects of drugs because of the following conditions that develop as part of the aging process.

1. The efficiency of all body systems declines. The ability of the liver and kidneys to metabolize and excrete drugs is less. The normal process of drug absorption, distribution in the body, and excretion from the body slows down. Therefore, dosages of certain drugs, such as for heart disease or control of psychotic behavior, are much less.

2. The elderly person may have several physical problems which call for administration of different-type drugs that may produce more symptoms if a careful analysis is not done. For instance, if a person needs heart medication that has a side effect of slowing down an electrical conduction in the heart, and the heart disease present is already doing the same thing, extreme care must be given to administering that drug.

3. Because of multiple conditions in a person at the same time, medication given for one diagnosis can cancel out the effects of medication for a second diagnosis. Drug interactions become a real problem.

The patterns of drug use are pronounced in the United States. Because of the heavy commercialization and promotion of drugs through the television media, over-the-counter (OTC) drug buying is heavy. The greatest number of people buying OTC drugs are those 65 years and older. The drugs bought most frequently upon prescription are those for the following conditions: heart disease, hypertension, arthritis, mental disorders, gastrointestinal problems, urinary tract infections, diabetes, coughs, sore throat, flu, circulatory problems, and chronic skin disorders. The institutionalized elderly use many more mind-altering drugs than the elderly living in the community. The reasons for these drugs are to combat depression, schizophrenia, and other mental disorders.

Common side effects of the mind-altering drugs include a drop in blood pressure, depression, confusion, agitation, hallucinations, constipation, dry mouth, difficulty urinating, hypothermia (drop in body temperature), and cardiac decompensation. Other side effects can include the condition *tardive dyskinesia*, which produces involuntary tongue movements, facial grimaces, and finger/arm and toe/leg movements. Over a long period of time, these movements can become irreversible.

The geriatric nursing assistant who gives the most care on a daily basis can detect obvious changes in behavior. These changes in behavior may be due to: a new drug, results of drug accumulation in the person's body of an old drug, or reactions to a combination of drugs. It is the responsibility of the geriatric nursing assistant to report these behavioral changes so that the licensed staff can investigate the causes. Behavior can change dramatically when a drug causing the behavior is stopped. Side effects may result in complications such as: fluid imbalance due to diarrhea, falls due to drop in blood pressure, and severe constipation due to dryness and loss of tone in the bowel. Disorientation and confusion can be the first signs of a drug reaction.

Figure 13.7 will help the geriatric nursing assistant to be alert for certain signs, symptoms, and behaviors. It is not necessary to know the exact medications the residents are taking, but knowing the category will help to determine if symptoms and changes in behavior are drug related.

Drug Category	Possible Effects
Analgesics: aspirin	Skin rash, diarrhea, constipation, ringing in the ears, deafness, bleeding tendency
Antidepressants (tricyclics): Elavil, Tofranil, Norpramin	Difficulty urinating, constipation, dry mouth, glaucoma, full-blown psychoses, agitation worsened
Antidepressants (MAO inhibitors): Nardil, Parnate (must control food)	Severe headache, hypertension crisis, nausea, vomiting, fever, chest pain, muscle twitching; no cheese, beer, and other products
Antidepressants (neuroleptic): Thorazine, Mellaril, Stelazine	Parkinsonia symptoms: rigid body, shuffle, drooling, motor restlessness; Tardive dyskinesa: curling of the tongue, facial grimaces, finger/arm and toe/leg movements, lip smacking
Antihypertensives: Aldomet, Serpasil	Headaches, dizziness, low blood pressure drop, drowsiness, sweating, dizziness
Antihistamines: Benadryl	Drowsiness, constipation, blurred vision, nervousness, excitement
Diuretics: Lasix	General weakness, nervousness, dehydration
Cardiac Medications: digitalis	Pulse below 60 per minute, nausea, vomiting, blurred vision, anorexia
Narcotics: morphine, demerol	Decreased respirations, delayed responses, oversedation
Sedatives: Valium, barbiturates	Excessive drowsiness, slurred speech, excessive excitability, increased restlessness, rage, falls, dizziness

Figure 13.7. Possible drug reactions to report.

KEY POINTS

1. Drugs and their administration are not the responsibility of nursing assistants; however, knowing what to watch for may help to prevent a crisis situation.
2. Many residents on drugs for high blood pressure are prone to falling. Take precautions by slowly getting these residents to change positions from lying or sitting to standing.
3. Confusion can be caused by drug interactions; report any confusion that suddenly occurs or is unexpected in a resident.

SELF-CHECK

1. A surgical opening in the trachea is called _____ .
2. Identify five nursing responses that an assistant can provide for a resident who has a new tracheostomy.

3. State the purpose of oxygen therapy.

4. Identify five geriatric nursing assistant responses for a person receiving oxygen by nasal cannula.

5. State why casts and traction are used.

6. Identify five geriatric nursing assistant responses for an elderly person in a wet cast.

7. Identify five geriatric nursing assistant responses for an elderly person in right-leg traction.

8. Mrs. White has high blood pressure. She receives medications which include a diuretic daily. She had to void just after breakfast. You were helping her to the bathroom when she felt dizzy and started to fall. (Look at the drug list.) What symptoms might be drug related? What will you report?

SUGGESTED ACTIVITIES

1. Visit a central supply department at a rehabilitation center or a hospital and ask to see the equipment used for tracheostomies, making casts, and setting up traction.
2. Visit hospital units and seek permission to visit patients who are using walled oxygen from a central supply, and patients who are in traction.
3. Talk with relatives and friends who have taken some of the medications on the checklist. Ask them about any reactions or side effects to the medication.
4. Speak to a pharmacist about drug side effects of patients.

CLINICAL APPLICATION

Using the problem-solving worksheet provided, select residents with the special therapies: tracheostomy, oxygen, casts, traction, and drugs, and apply geriatric nursing assistant responses.

WORKSHEET

Nursing Responses: Tracheostomy

Resident: _____   Diagnosis: _____
       (first name only)

Description of the therapy: (Briefly describe the type of therapy as it pertains to this unit.)

Geriatric Nursing Assistant Responses:
Needs   Nursing Responses

Progress after nursing responses:

WORKSHEET

Nursing Responses: Oxygen

Resident: _____   Diagnosis: _____
      (first name only)

Description of the therapy: (Briefly describe the type of therapy as it pertains to this unit.)

Geriatric Nursing Assistant Responses:
Needs   Nursing Responses

Progress after nursing responses:

WORKSHEET

Nursing Responses: Casts

Resident: _____   Diagnosis: _____
          (first name only)

Description of the therapy: (Briefly describe the type of therapy as it pertains to this unit.)

Geriatric Nursing Assistant Responses:
Needs   Nursing Responses
_____   _____

Progress after nursing responses:

WORKSHEET

Nursing Responses: Traction

Resident: _____   Diagnosis: _____
      (first name only)

Description of the therapy: (Briefly describe the type of therapy as it pertains to this unit.)

Geriatric Nursing Assistant Responses:
Needs   Nursing Responses

Progress after nursing responses:

WORKSHEET

Nursing Responses: Drugs

Resident: _____   Diagnosis: _____
      (first name only)

Description of the therapy: (Briefly describe the type of therapy as it pertains to this unit.)

Geriatric Nursing Assistant Responses:

Needs   Nursing Responses

Progress after nursing responses:

14 REDUCING JOB-RELATED STRESS

TERMINAL PERFORMANCE OBJECTIVE

Given information on stress and stress factors related to the job as a geriatric nursing assistant, be able to develop a personal plan of stress management, which will reduce stress on the job as a geriatric nursing assistant.

Enabling Objectives

1. Define the concept of stress.
2. Identify five types of stressors.
3. Identify techniques for coping with stress.
4. Define time management.
5. Identify five considerations in managing personal time.
6. Identify five factors to be considered in a personal stress control plan.
7. Develop a personal plan of stress control which includes time management and will reduce stress related to the job.

REVIEW SECTION

The geriatric nursing assistant should review with the instructor how stress contributes to disease and how its meaning differs for each person.

THE CONCEPT OF STRESS

The concept of stress has been the center of much research in the last few years. There has been a heightened awareness of stress in the form of books, journals, news media publications, and in the presentation of workshops for the management of stress. Writers from many disciplines, such as medicine, psychology, and sociology, have contributed to the understanding and to the confusion of the concept. However, each of us has a good idea of what stress is because we have had it at one time or another. Each person feels stress in a different way, which adds to the mystery of the concept.

According to Dr. Hans Selye, a pioneering researcher in the field, no matter what causes stress in people, there is an identical biological stress reaction called the *general adaptation syndrome*. Dr. Selye has described three stages as part of the syndrome which helps our bodies to respond to the demand that the agent of the stress (the stressor) puts upon us. Our bodies must adapt to the stressor and return to its normal or nearly normal state, called *homeostasis*. In the first stage of the adaptation syndrome, called the *alarm reaction*, hormones are activated and these summon our bodies' defenses. Perhaps you remember a time when you were frightened and your heart started to pound, your pulse rate increased, and your body tightened. These feelings were caused by hormones working on key organs of the body. If the agent of stress becomes less threatening, the second phase of the syndrome takes over. In this stage, called *resistance*, the hormones' activity is reversed. If homeostasis is not reached and the body does not return to normal, the third phase of exhaustion takes over until the body depletes itself, and death occurs.

The first two stages, Dr. Selye says, are experienced many times over. The agents, or stressors, can be physical, such as a bacterium that causes a disease; or psychological, such as fear. Stress can also be good, such as joy or happiness. When the agent is seen by the person as bad, distress occurs. When the agent is seen as good, eustress occurs. (See the later list of definitions for further explanation of terms.)

If the state of stress is prolonged and increases in intensity, disease can occur. Dr. Selye has listed the most common diseases due to stress as diseases of adaptation: peptic ulcers, high blood pressure, heart attacks, and nervous disorders. He cautioned that these diseases do not exclude the influence of other factors, such as a person having a genetic predisposition to a defective organ or having had a previous disease in the organ involved. If additional factors are within a person, there is more risk of developing the disease.

Other researchers have recognized the pioneering work of Dr. Selye but have emphasized that the difference in individual responses to stressors has to do with how the person perceives the stressful agent and how he or she appraises the demand expected. In other words, what is stressful to one person may be quite different, even joyful, to another person (Figure 14.1).

A central idea that is being researched is how people cope with different stressors. Why is it some people have many stresses in their lives and rarely succumb to illness while others are always ill? Some researchers have said that experience with stress helps a person to diminish the effects of another stressor.

There is much controversy and doubt and a lot of research going on about how people overcome stress and how stress actually relates to disease. Research, for instance, has confirmed that people who have a Type A personality are very prone to coronary heart disease.

Other research has shown that as people age, their immune systems decline and they become more susceptible to disease. Researchers envision that at some time in the future treatment of the immune system will possibly effect retardation of the aging process and the disease process.

That there is a connection between stress and disease seems very obvious. An area of agreement among some physicians, psychologists, and sociologists is that to explain any disease process, the professionals must take into account psychological factors, including responses to environmental stress, and mechanisms used to cope with the stress.

The abundance of research indicates that there are many factors involved in trying to reach an agreement on how stress relates to, or contributes to the cause of, disease; *however, there is a definite relationship.*

DEFINITIONS OF TERMS RELATED TO STRESS

Stress: "nonspecific response of the body to any demand made upon it" (Selye).

Distress: damaging or unpleasant stress (Selye).

Eustress: less damaging wear and tear because the stimulus is reasoned to be pleasant and not a threat (Selye).

Homeostasis: coordinated physiological processes which maintain most of the steady states in the organism (Selye).

Coping: To deal with and attempt to overcome problems and difficulties (*Webster's*); efforts to manage environmental stimuli and internal demands and conflicts among demands (Lazarus).

Stressors: situations, agents, or stimuli that result in stress reactions; any stimulus that results in wear and tear on the body.

DIAGRAMMATIC VIEW OF STRESS REACTION

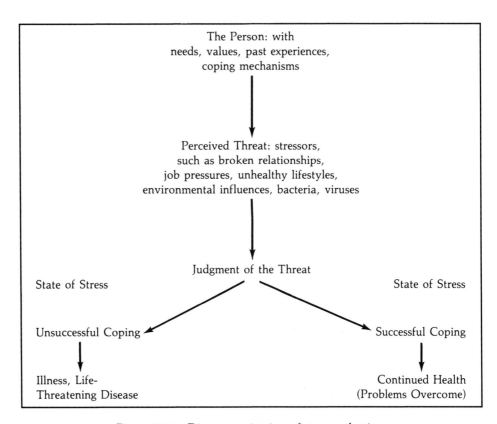

Figure 14.1. Diagrammatic view of stress reduction.

STRESS CONTROL TEST*

The following test contains factors known to enhance ability to deal with stress.

Directions: Read the following statements and circle either yes or no.

I eat a balanced diet every day.	Yes	No
I am sure to get 8 hours of sleep 4 to 5 days a week.	Yes	No
I drink 6 to 8 glasses of water daily.	Yes	No
I exchange affection (hugging) daily.	Yes	No
I exercise 30 to 40 minutes three times a week.	Yes	No
I smoke less than one pack of cigarettes a day.	Yes	No
I do not smoke or am I trying to quit smoking.	Yes	No
I do not drink alcohol excessively.	Yes	No
I am not overweight for my height and bone structure.	Yes	No
I have enough income to meet my basic needs.	Yes	No
I attend a church of my choice regularly.	Yes	No
I attend social activities and participate in diversional activities regularly.	Yes	No
I have a relative I can rely on within 50 miles from me.	Yes	No
I have someone with whom I can confide on matters of importance.	Yes	No
I am in good health (including eyesight, hearing, and teeth).	Yes	No
I am able to speak openly about my feelings when angry or worried.	Yes	No
I have regular conversations with the people I live with about chores, money, and daily living issues.	Yes	No
I do something for fun at least once per week.	Yes	No
I organize my time at home and on the job effectively.	Yes	No
I drink less than 3 cups of caffeinated beverages daily.	Yes	No
I find adequate quiet time for myself daily.	Yes	No

Count the number of "yes" answers. Ideally, they should all be "yes." The more "yes" answers, the less vulnerable you are to stress in your life.

COPING

One of the definitions given on the list of definitions for the word *coping* is: "to deal with and attempt to overcome problems and difficulties." The process of coping, as in the concept of stress, is highly individual. However, researchers have given us some suggestions on how to manage the stresses in our lives, how best to cope.

Dr. Hans Selye, one of the most honored researchers, gave this advice:

* Find your own stress level—work as hard as you like as long as it is natural for you.
* Establish a goal in life and strive to attain it as long as in your achievement you gain the esteem and goodwill of others.

*From L. Miller, cited in the *Bostonian*, Boston University, Boston, MA.

Other experts offer the following guidelines:

1. Find a meaning and purpose in life.
2. Build a personal support system of family and friends: Verbalize your frustrations.
3. Watch your intake of:
   a. Saturated fats
   b. Refined sugars and starches
   c. Caffeine-loaded products
   d. Alcohol and other drugs that are addicting
4. Get exercise.
5. Use relaxing techniques.
6. Seek good information when needed for solving problems.

Coping with stress: a summary

1. Problem solve—identify the problem.
2. Get help—have a listener.
3. Socialize—talk it out with co-workers; decide what can be done; and then change the subject.
4. Develop assertive skills.
5. Set priorities—manage life and responsibilities.
6. Appreciate others—let them know it.
7. Take a short vacation.
8. Vary the job.
9. Practice relaxation techniques.
10. Participate in physical activity.
11. Develop outside interests.

Stress has such a personal nature to it that only the person having the stress can alter the consequences. Steps in resolving the stress are considered by most experts to include the following:

1. Identify personal feelings and the circumstances that are causing the stress: diagnose the problem.
2. Seek information that will help to resolve the situation and find coping mechanisms to deal with it.
3. Apply what is learned to everyday life.

STRESSORS RELATED TO THE JOB

In the role of geriatric nursing assistant, stress can build because of daily interactions and communications with staff and residents. This section refers primarily to interactions with staff. The unit on communication concentrated on how to relate to residents. The tendency is to blame another person for making us feel badly about what he or she said. There are some techniques that can help counter stress due to statements that hurt our feelings. The first step is to change a personal attitude about the statement.

Statement: The charge nurse reprimands you because you spilled a cup of coffee.

Your thoughts:	The charge nurse thinks I'm stupid; she doesn't like me anyway. I'm just a klutz.
Personal reaction:	I feel awful; I'll never amount to anything. She will never like me. I won't get the raise in pay I need.

Resolving stressful situations brought on by communication can be helped by thinking through what brought on your reaction. Was your thinking rational? Ask other people if they would agree with your thinking. Probably they would not. Your thoughts could be called irrational. To overcome the irrationality of your thinking follow these steps:

1. Decide if your thoughts are rational.
2. Change your attitude about your thoughts and feelings. In this situation you learn to reverse the feelings. An example is the following: "The charge nurse never said I was stupid or a klutz. Other people drop coffee cups. I didn't hurt anybody when I did it. I'll wipe it up." The sooner you can talk sense to yourself, the quicker the stress will leave.

This process of reversing the irrational way of thinking and feeling helps to eliminate the stress caused by the feelings of inadequacy and "I'll never amount to anything." In their book *Talk Sense to Yourself*, McMillen and Casey offer ways to talk to yourself to rid yourself of irrational thoughts:

1. This thought only hurts me. What good is all the pain? It changes nothing and only makes me feel bad.
2. This thought is a great way to lose friends.
3. This thought is pointless. It doesn't get me any closer to my goals.
4. This thought has absolutely nothing to do with reality. It just ain't so!

Using the technique listed above is one way of getting rid of the thoughts that nag you. Another way to counter negative feelings in interactions is with the use of assertive techniques. If you find you really cannot express what you feel, assertiveness training is recommended. Using assertive statements can help eliminate the feelings that cause stress.

Note: It must be remembered that these suggestions are for use when interacting with staff members and not with residents. Residents may say things that are very unkind because of mental deterioration. Geriatric nursing assistants must consider the resident's mental and physical condition when responding to unkind remarks.

Assertive statements allow you to say "I feel, I want, I need, and I am (angry, happy, confused). *It is important to remember that you, and only you, control your feelings.* You can really think your way out of feeling badly if you apply rational thoughts based on assertive techniques. Assertive behavior originates with how we perceive ourselves. It is possible to tell someone "I am furious" when you are angry because of something they did or said. In this way you express your feelings without hurting the other person with, "You are the cause of my anger, you are stupid!" With the first expression, you allow the other person to think about how they contributed to your feelings. Another major factor that may cause a lot of stress on the job is time. Managing one's time effectively can reduce the amount of stress.

TIME MANAGEMENT

Time management is defined as making the most efficient use of your time. In this case it means making the most efficient use of your time within the shift you are working. Time management begins with planning and organizing the time during which you will be working so that the priorities of your responsibilities are met. Priority setting should begin with the residents to whom you are assigned. The residents are the most important responsibility; without them you would not be working.

You can begin priority setting by learning your assignment and making rounds with the offgoing and oncoming nursing care teams. In this way you can identify who will need what kinds of care first. Priority setting means determining what must be done first, second, third, and so on.

The geriatric nursing assistant will have other responsibilities which are not directly involved in care of residents. These responsibilities will involve such duties as cleaning, taking care of dirty laundry, and charting. Having a work schedule will help the nursing assistant to keep a record of times and responsibilities and have a plan to write notes for charting (see Figure 14.2).

Thinking and working as a team member and sharing responsibilities will help to make the work involved become more efficient. For example, knowing what kind of assistance might be needed to transfer residents must be considered and done cooperatively with other nursing assistants. As a geriatric nursing team member, you can assist someone else when he or she needs assistance with respon-

Time	Residents	Nursing Responses	Evaluation	Other Duties
0700	Mr. Jones	Prepare breakfast AM care	Ate full breakfast	
	Ms. Smith	Out of bed with help; AM care	Ate 50%; bathed self; assisted with hair care	
0800	Mr. Brown	To x-ray, then shower		Stock linen cart
	Ms. White	Assist with AM care; take vital signs	150/90 98.8-68-22	
0900	Ms. White	To P.T.	Refused, feeling nauseated; reported to charge nurse	
1000 1100 up to 3:00pm				

Evaluation of the day: What could be done better? What worked effectively? What interfered with my original plan for the day:

Figure 14.2.   Sample worksheet for time management on the job.

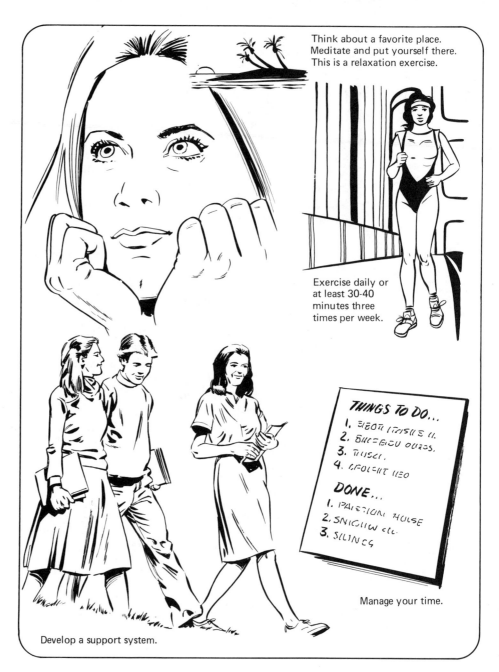

Think about a favorite place.
Meditate and put yourself there.
This is a relaxation exercise.

Exercise daily or
at least 30-40
minutes three
times per week.

THINGS TO DO...

DONE...

Manage your time.

Develop a support system.

Figure 14.3. Be good to yourself.

sibilities. A good team member is available to help others when there is time to spare. Incorporating a time to reflect and evaluate your shift will help to discover ways to improve the next day and to reduce the stress that occurs when time is running out.

There are other considerations when thinking about time management. Are you a morning person, someone who likes to get up early and get started right away? Or are you a night person, someone who does a lot of work late in the evening? It may be that your hardest chores should be saved for late evening or early morning, depending on when you are most efficient. If you are being told by your supervisor that you are lazy or don't work fast enough, it could be due to the shift you work. You might want to change shifts to be more productive at a time when your energy level is highest.

If there is a great deal of stress in your life, develop a stress control plan and do something about controlling the stressors (Figure 14.3). A guide for a stress control plan follows. A Daily Time Manager worksheet has also been provided for daily use (Figure 14.4). It will help to organize your activities away

DAILY TIME MANAGER

Date: _____ Day _____				
Priority#	People to Call/Number		Time	Appointments
Priority#	Letters to Write		Shopping List	
Priority#	Things to Do		Miscellaneous Activities	
	Reward myself with: Exercise by:			

Remember: Do your hardest chores when you have the most energy. Mark through activities when they are completed. Exercise and reward yourself.

Figure 14.4. Daily time manager.

from the job. Prioritizing your activities each day will help you to use time more efficiently. You will also feel better when you check off what you have accomplished for the day.

A STRESS CONTROL PLAN

Directions: Stress control requires that you start doing something about it. Use this plan to begin stress control today.

1. Identify stressors by making a list of the pressures that produce stress in you. (What do others do that cause you to become upset?)

2. Identify the things you do that cause stress in others. (Maybe you constantly "nag" someone about a bad habit, or you smoke and no one else does.)

3. Go over steps 1 and 2 to see if there are some things you can change as the days go by.

4. Now write down something that *you have been neglecting to do* and do it before the day is over. (Write to your mother, or call a friend, or whatever you keep forgetting to do.)

5. Write down the name of someone close to you and something specific you will do for that person today.

6. Write down something special you will do for yourself today.

7. Consider other factors that cause stress and decide on a goal which will help to relieve the stress. (Perhaps it will mean gathering information to help make a decision.)

8. Establish a goal that will help you physically as well as emotionally (a daily bike ride, walking, swimming, etc.).

9. If you are concerned about another person, plan how you will go about working out these concerns with that person.

10. Review your daily activities and the energy you expend. When do you accomplish the most? (Are you a morning person or a night person?) You should consider doing those things that require the most energy during the peak times of your energy level.

11. Look at your daily schedule and redo it to meet the responsibilities so you will have the energy to do them. *Don't procrastinate. Don't put off.* The nagging thought of things undone causes stress.

12. Be good to yourself. Remember you cannot change everything—it is knowing the difference between what you can and cannot change that will help you conquer stress.

KEY POINTS

1. Most care givers at some time or other begin to feel "burned out." A restoration period is necessary when this happens. Suggestions have been provided to help you to "refill your cup" of good feelings about those for whom you care and about yourself.

2. It is okay to tell people how you feel when what they say and do hurts you. Take assertiveness training.
3. Everyone needs a support system of people to help when the going gets rough. Make that a priority. A support system is a coping mechanism for stress.
4. Managing your time on the job will help reduce stress.
5. Maybe rearranging to do difficult tasks when your energy level is high will reduce stress in your life.
6. Develop a personal stress plan. Being a geriatric nursing assistant can be very stressful at times. It is okay to admit that. It is not okay to do nothing about it.

SUGGESTED ACTIVITIES

1. Learn relaxation exercises.
2. Design a personal stress-reducing activity.
3. Share your stress-reducing activities with your relatives and friends. Help them to reduce stress in their lives.

CLINICAL APPLICATION

Using the information in this unit, develop a personal stress control plan, and share the information and the plan with your co-workers. Initiate stress control at your place of work.

READING LIST

BURNSIDE, I.M. (1988). *Nursing and the aged.* 3rd. ed. New York: McGraw-Hill.

BOWKER, L.H. (1982). *Humanizing institutions for the aged.* Lexington, MA : D.C. Heath.

BUTLER, R.N. (1975). *Why survive! Being old in America.* New York : Harper and Row.

CHENITZ, W. C. (1985). Entry into a nursing home as status passage: A theory to guide nursing practice. *Geriatric Nursing,* March/April: 92–97.

COUSINS, N. (1979). *Anatomy of an illness.* Toronto : W.W. Norton.

MATTESON, M.A. AND McCONNELL, E.S. (1988). *Gerontological Nursing.* Philadelphia, PA: W.B. Saunders Co.

McMULLIN, R. AND CASEY, B. (1975). *Talk sense to yourself.* Lakewood, CO: Jefferson County Mental Health Center, Inc.

SMITH, P.W. (1984). *Infection control in long term care facilities.* New York : John Wiley and Sons, Inc.

WILL, C.A. AND EIGHMY, B. (1988). *Being a long-term care nursing assistant.* 2nd ed. Englewood Cliffs, NJ: Prentice-Hall (A Brady Book).

GLOSSARY

Abduction To move an arm or leg away from the center of the body.

Acute-sharp Course of short duration (as with disease); most severe part of illness.

Accuracy Factual or being correct.

Acetone Byproduct of the metabolism of fat; a type of ketone.

Activities of Daily Living (ADL) Activities or tasks needed for daily living, such as eating, grooming, dressing, bathing, washing, and toileting.

Adduction To move an arm or leg toward the center of the body.

Adrenal Glands Two small glands located on top of each kidney, producing hormones that help the body react and adapt to stress.

AIDS Acquired immunodeficiency syndrome.

Alignment To put in a straight line.

Alveoli Tiny air sacs in the lungs where oxygen enters the blood.

Alzheimer's Disease (AD) A disease of mental deterioration.

Ambulation Walking or moving about in an upright position.

Ambulation Device Any apparatus to assist with walking, includes braces, canes, crutches, and walkers.

Amino Acids The units of structure in proteins.

Analgesics Medications that relieve pain.

Anatomy Study of body parts, how the body is made, and what it is made of.

Aneurysm Bulging out of the wall of an artery.

Anterior In front of.

Antibiotics Medications that treat acute infections; they inhibit the growth of disease-producing organisms.

Antidepressants Medications used to combat depressive states.

Antihistamines Medications used to combat allergies.

Anxiety A feeling of worry and uneasiness.

Aorta Largest artery in the body.

Aphasia Loss of language or communication ability.

Apical Pulse Heartbeat measured at the apex of the heart.

Apnea Absence of breathing.

Arteries Blood vessels that carry blood away from the heart.

Arterioles Tiny arteries that carry blood from the large arteries to the capillaries.

Arteriosclerosis Thickening, hardening, and loss of elasticity in the arteries.

Arthritis Inflammation of a joint.

Aseptic Free of microorganisms.

Aspiration Inhaling food or fluid into the lungs.

Assertiveness Expressing feelings without violating the rights of others.

Assessment The act of gathering facts to identify needs and problems.

Atherosclerosis Clogging of the inner lining of the arteries with plaque and deposits of calcium or fat.

Atrophy Decreasing of muscle mass; wasting of muscle tissue.

Autoclaving Method of sterilization using pressurized steam.

Autoimmune Disease A disease resulting from the body's immune system reacting against its own body parts.

Autonomic Nervous System Part of the nervous system that controls organs not under conscious control.

Axillary In the armpit.

Back Blows Rapid series of sharp whacks delivered with the hand over the spine between the shoulder blades.

Bacterium Singular of bacteria, a type of microorganism.

Behaving Courteously Putting the needs of others before your own.

Benign Prostatic Hypertrophy Noncancerous enlargement of the prostate gland.

Bile Substance stored in the gallbladder that aids in the digestion of fats.

Biopsy Excision of a small piece of tissue.

Blood Pressure Measurable force of the blood against the walls of a blood vessel.

Body Mechanics Ways of standing and moving one's body.

Bronchi Two main branches of the windpipe.

Bursa Small fluid-filled sac that allows one bone to move easily over another bone.

Bursitis Inflammation of the fluid-filled sacs, causing pain on movement.

Cancer Form of cellular disorder in which the normal mechanisms of the cell (that control rate of growth, cell division, and movement) are disrupted.

Capillaries Smallest blood vessels in the circulatory system. They nourish body cells.

Cardiac Muscle Tissue Type of muscle tissue in the heart that controls the heartbeat.

Caring Compassion; understanding the fears, problems, and distress of another.

Cartilage Tough gristle-like substance that forms a pad at the end of or between bones.

Cataracts Eye lenses that are clouded.

Cauterize To burn, as with tissue, with a hot iron or chemicals.

CC Cubic centimeters; a liquid measurement equal to milliliters (ml).

Cell Fundamental building block of all living organisms.

Cell Membrane Rim or edge of the cell.

Center of Gravity Place where the bulk or mass of an object is centered.

Cerebellum Part of the brain that coordinates voluntary movement.

Cerebrovascular Accident (CVA) Stroke.

Cerebrospinal Fluid Fluid in the central nervous system.

Cerebrum Part of the brain responsible for thinking, learning, and memory.

Chart Written health or medical record, which is a legal document.

Chemotherapy Use of drugs or medications to treat disease.

Cheyne-Stoke's Respirations Irregular breathing; periods of apnea, and periods of deep breathing; associated with a person who is dying.

Chronic Of long duration.

Cilia Small hair-like projections of the respiratory passages.

Cirrhosis Inflammation of a tissue or organ, particularly the liver.

Clean Uncontaminated; free from known pathogenic organisms.

Code of Ethics Rules of conduct for a particular group.

Collagen   A fibrous protein found in skin and bone.

Communicable Conditions   Diseases and infections that spread from one person to another.

Communication   Involves a sender, a message, a medium, a receiver and feedback; involves speaking or writing, or facial expressions, tone of voice, gestures, body position, and movement.

Complete Airway Obstruction   Blocking of the airway so that no air passes through.

Confidentiality   Not revealing private information to others.

Confused   Not oriented to self, time, or place.

Congestive Heart Failure   Inability of the heart to pump out all the blood returned to it from the veins.

Connective Tissue   Tissue that connects and supports other tissue.

Conjunctivitis   Inflammation of the conjunctiva of the eye.

Constipation   Buildup of fecal material in the large intestine.

Contaminated   Not sterile; in contact with microorganisms.

Continuity   Doing the same thing in the same way.

Contracture   Permanent shortening of the muscle, leading to permanent disability or loss of function.

Convulsions   Jerking of the muscles as they contract and relax.

Counter-Traction   Exertion of pull in the opposite direction of traction.

Cranium   The skull or bones of the head.

Creutzfeldt-Jakob Disease   An incurable disease of the central nervous system.

Cultural   Beliefs and social forms of a racial, religious or social group.

Cyanosis   Blue or gray color of the skin, lips, and nailbeds, indicating lack of oxygen.

Cystitis   Inflammation of the urinary bladder.

Debridement   Removal of dead or unhealthy tissue.

Decibel   Unit of measurement used in determining hearing loss.

Decubitus Ulcers   Tissue breakdown resulting from pressure or reduced blood flow (often called pressure sores or bed sores); also called decubiti when there is more than one.

Defecation   Process of elimination of waste material from the bowel.

Deficit   A deficiency or loss.

Dehydration   Condition in which fluid output is greater than fluid intake.

Dementia   Mental deterioration.

Depression   Mental condition involving lack of interest in usual activities.

Dermis   Second layer of the skin.

Dermatitis   Inflammation of the skin.

Diabetes Mellitus   Disease in which the pancreas secretes insufficient amounts of insulin.

Diabetic Coma   High blood sugar with presence of ketone in the urine.

Diaphragm   Muscular organ that separates the chest and abdominal cavities.

Diarrhea   Semi-fluid feces.

Diplomatic   Skilled in relationships.

Dirty   Contaminated, used or exposed to disease-producing organisms.

Disability   Limitation in the ability to function normally.

Disinfection   Process of killing most microorganisms.

Diuretics   Medications used to promote fluid excretion.

Diverticulum   A sac or pouch in wall of an organ.

Documentation   Writing appropriately and accurately the facts of a situation.

Dorsiflexion   To flex the ankle (away from the sole of the foot).

DRG   Diagnostic related group.

Duodenum   First loop of the small intestine.

Dyspnea   Difficulty breathing.

Edema Swelling of joints, tissue, or organs.

Edentulousness Tooth loss.

Ego The self.

Ego Strength The strength of a person's ego as perceived by the person; associated with a person's sense of self-esteem.

Ejaculation Ejection of seminal fluid from the male urethra.

Elderly People over 65 years of age.

Electrolytes Solutions containing substances that conduct electricity: sodium, potassium, chloride.

Electrocardiagram Tracing of the heart's electrical conduction system.

Embolus A blood clot that moves within the blood stream.

Emotional Reaction of the emotions, for example, crying or laughing.

Empathy Ability to put yourself in another's place and to see things as they do.

Enema Introduction of fluid into the rectum and colon.

Environmentally Pertains to the surroundings.

Epidemiologic Relates to the study of disease and how it is distributed in populations.

Epidermis Outer layer of the skin.

Epiglottis Cartilage which covers the opening of the trachea when foods and fluids are swallowed.

Erythema Redness of the skin.

Estrogen Female sex hormone.

Exacerbation Return of symptoms.

Excoriated Redness and abrasion of the skin.

Extension To straighten an arm or leg.

Exudate Drainage of fluid, pus, serum.

Fallopian Tubes Tubes from the ovary to the uterus through which the ovum passes.

Feces Solid human waste.

Finger Probes Manual removal of a foreign body by using the index finger.

Fluid Balance The individual takes in and eliminates about the same amount of fluid.

Fluid Intake Total amount of fluid taken into the body over a given amount of time.

Fluid Output Total amount of fluid eliminated from the body in a given amount of time.

Force (Pulse) Strength or power described as weak or bounding.

Fracture Breaking or cracking of a bone.

Friedreich's Ataxia Inherited degenerative disease of the spinal cord.

Functioning Ability The ability to perform; usually refers to activities of daily living.

Gastritis Inflammation of the stomach caused by many different factors.

Gatch Handle or crank used to raise and lower the bed, head of bed or foot of bed.

Geriatric Pertaining to care and treatment of the aging.

Glaucoma Eye disease with pressure in the eye and leads to nerve damage and blindness.

Glomerulus A network of capillaries in the kidney that filters the blood.

Glucose Simple sugar.

Glycosuria Sugar in the urine.

Gravity Attraction that the earth has for an object on or near its surface.

Heart Muscle that pumps blood through the vessels.

Hemiplegia Paralysis of one side of the body.

Hemorrhoids Enlarged blood-filled vessels that surround the rectal area.

Hiatal Hernia Part of stomach rises through the opening of the diaphragm.

HIV Human immunodeficiency virus.

Holistic Total interacting parts; more than the sum of the parts.

Home Health Care Agencies Businesses that provide health services to clients in the home.

Homeostasis   Body's attempt to keep its internal environment stable and in balance.

Humanistic   Pertaining to human interaction and a value for dignity and worth of each person.

Huntington's Disease   Inherited disease of the brain and nervous system with early life onset.

Hydrochloric Acid   Acid in the stomach.

Hyperextension   To move beyond the normal extension.

Hyperglycemia   High blood sugar.

Hyperthermia   Body temperature of 105 degrees Farenheit or more.

Hypostatic Pneumonia   Pneumonia due to blood stagnation in one part of the lung.

Hypotension   Low blood pressure.

Hypothalamus   Gland in the brain that controls body temperature and the function of the endocrine glands.

Hypothermia   Body temperature of 95 degrees Farenheit or less.

Hypothyroidism   Decreased production of thyroid hormone.

Imbalance   Lack of equality or equilibrium.

Implement   To carry out or accomplish a given plan.

Impotence   Inability to engage in sexual intercourse.

Incident Report   Written description of an accident involving resident, visitor or staff member.

Incontinent   No control over bowel or bladder function.

Indwelling Catheter   Tube inserted into the bladder to drain urine into a collection bag.

Infarct   Death of part of the heart muscle.

Infection   Invasion of the body by a disease-producing organism.

Inferior   Toward the feet.

Inflammation   Tissue reaction to disease or injury characterized by heat, redness, pain, and swelling.

Influenza   Acute lung infection due to a virus.

Insulin   Hormone secreted by the pancreas.

Insulin Shock   Low blood sugar, usually from too much insulin or not enough food intake.

Invasion of Privacy   When personal information is exposed publicly, violating an individual's right to privacy.

Isolation   To separate or set apart.

Isolation Techniques   Safety measures to prevent spread of communicable conditions.

Job Description   Contains the duties of a particular job category.

Kyphosis   Hunchback or stooped curving of the thoracic spine.

Lactic Acid   Milky liquid formed by breakdown of glycogen in muscles.

Larynx   Voice box.

Laxative   Medication that loosens the bowel contents and encourages evacuation.

Legal   According to laws of the community, state, or nation.

Lens   The crystalline refracting medium of the eye.

Lifestyle   A person's way of life.

Ligaments   Tough, white, fibrous cords that connect bone to bone.

Lordosis   Abnormal anterior curvature of spine.

Lymph   Fluid which surrounds the body cells.

Lymph Vessels   Tiny capillary-like structures that collect lymph.

Macular Degeneration   Destruction of macula, part of the retina, and loss of central vision.

Making Rounds   Going to look at each resident to determine his or her immediate needs.

Malignant   Growing worse; used with cancerous condition.

Malnutrition   Poorly nourished.

Mammary Glands   Glandular tissue of the breast.

Manual Thrusts   Series of rapid thrusts to the upper abdomen or chest that force air from the lungs.

Medulla Vital center in the brain that controls breathing, swallowing, and heartbeat.

Metabolic Rate The rate of energy use.

Metabolism Complex processes of the living cells where oxygen is used and carbon dioxide is given off (called the work of the cell).

Metastasize Spread to other parts of the body.

Microorganisms Tiny living things seen only with a microscope.

Midbrain Part of the brain through which nerve impulses pass.

ML Milliliters, liquid measurement, equal to cubic centimeters (cc).

Moist Application Application where water touches the skin.

Morbidity Illness.

Mortality Death.

Multidisciplinary Team Professionals with different educational backgrounds who work together.

Multi-Infarct Dementia Brain deterioration due to many strokes.

Myocardial Infarction Heart attack in which part of the heart muscle dies.

Narcotics Medications that relieve pain; can be addicting.

Nasal Cannula Tube with openings that fit into each nare for administering oxygen.

Nausea Unpleasant sensation prior to vomiting.

Negligence Failure to act as an average nursing assistant would act under the same circumstances.

Nephrons Microscopic filtering units of the kidney.

Neurons Specialized cells of the nervous system.

Neurotransmitter A substance that helps to transmit messages between neurons.

Nocturia Need to get up at night to urinate.

Non-Pathogenic Not capable of producing disease.

Nonprofit Operated without profit or gain.

Nosocomial Pertains to infections which occur to a person while a patient in a hospital or health care facility.

Nutrition Science of food and its actions or relationship to health.

Objective Observations Facts observed and not distorted by personal feelings.

Observation Recognizing and noticing a fact or occurrence.

Obstruction Blocking of the airway.

Olfaction Sense of smell.

Optimal Most desirable.

Oral In the mouth.

Oral Hygiene Care of the mouth, teeth, gums, and tongue.

Organ Body part where two or more tissues work together to perform a particular function.

Organism Any living thing.

Orientation Ability to accurately describe person, place, and time.

Osteoarthritis Disease characterized by deterioration of joint cartilage and formation of new bone at joint surfaces.

Osteoporosis Disease characterized by porous or chalklike bones which fracture very easily.

Ostomy Surgical opening made on the surface of the abdomen to release waste from the body.

Ovaries Primary female reproductive organs.

Pancreas Large gland located in the abdomen; secretes insulin and glucagon.

Paralysis Loss of voluntary movement.

Paranoid Pertains to mental state where a person becomes suspicious and feels persecuted.

Paraplegic Person with paralysis of the lower limbs.

Parathyroid Glands Two pairs of glands located within the thyroid that produce a hormone to help regulate the level of calcium and phosphorus in the body.

Parkinson's Disease Degenerative disease of the nervous system.

Partial Airway Obstruction   Incomplete blocking of the airway, allowing some air to pass through.

Patency   Freely open.

Pathogenic   Causing disease.

Penis   Primary male sex organ.

Perinatal   Around the time of birth.

Peripheral Vascular Disease   Poor circulation in the extremities.

Peristalsis   Rhythmic contractions that assist in moving food through the intestines.

Personality   The totality of a person's behavior.

Philosophy   Beliefs and attitudes about individuals and groups.

Physical Needs   Basic human needs for food, water, oxygen, rest, exercise, and sexual activity; needs of the body.

Physiology   Study of how the body functions, how all the body parts work independently and collectively.

Pick's Disease   A disease of mental deterioration.

Pituitary Gland   Master gland of the body.

Plantar Flexion   Extending the ankle (toward the sole of the foot).

Pneumonia   Acute infection of the lung.

Policy   Describes what is to be done.

Pons   Part of the brain through which nerve impulses pass.

Posterior   In back of.

Postural Support   Soft protective device or restraint used to protect a person from injury.

Presbycusis   Hearing impairment related to aging.

Presbyopia   Visual impairment; can not see well up close.

Prerequisite   Required before, such as before taking a course of study.

Procedure   Description of how to do a task.

Prolapse   Protruding, such as the uterus into the vagina.

Pronation   Turning palms down.

Prosthesis   Artificial body part.

Pruritus   Severe itching.

Psychological   Relates to the mind and mental activity.

Psychosocial   Referring to an individual's mental or emotional processes, in combination with their ability to interact and relate with others.

Pulse Rate   Number of pulse beats per minute.

Pulse Rhythm   Regularity of the pulse beats.

Pyelonephritis   Inflammation of the pelvis of the kidney.

Radial Deviation   Toward the thumb side of the hand.

Radial Pulse   Pulse felt at the inner aspect of the wrist (radial artery).

Range of Motion   Extent to which a joint can be moved through its usual actions before causing pain.

Rapport   Respect and understanding between two or more people.

Reality Orientation   Technique for reducing or eliminating disorientation.

Rectal   In the rectum.

Rectum   Lowest section of the large intestine adjacent to the outside of the body.

Rehabilitation   Regaining a state of health; helping residents do as much as they can, as well as they can, for as long as they can.

Rehabilitation Philosophy   Belief which promotes independence and recognizes the accomplishment of reaching goals, short term and long term.

Reflex   Automatic response to stimulation.

Re-Infection   Being infected a second time.

Remission   Lessening or disappearance of disease symptoms.

Renal Artery   Artery that supplies blood to the kidneys.

Respect   Recognizing and showing the worth of another person.

Respiration   Process of inhaling and exhaling.

Restraint   Object that holds back; used in reference to postural support or soft protective devices.

Rheumatoid Arthritis   Disease characterized by painful, stiff, swollen red joints that eventually become deformed.

Role   Part one plays in relationship to others.

Rotation   To move a joint in a circular motion around its axis.

Salivary Glands   Glands that produce saliva to moisten the mouth and begin the digestion of food.

Scalpel   Surgical knife.

Scrotum   Sac outside the male containing the testes.

Security Needs   Basic human needs for physical safety, shelter, protection.

Sedatives   Medications to calm and produce sleep.

Self-Actualization   A person has all needs satisfied; occurs in adulthood.

Self-Fulfillment   Basic human need to reach the highest potential and to accomplish one's life goals; self-actualization.

Semen   Fluid expelled through the penis during ejaculation; contains sperm, water and nutrients.

Senility   Mental and physical weakness of old age.

Sensitivity   Ability to detect or respond.

Septum   Tissue which divides the heart into right and left chambers.

Sexuality   Quality of being male or female.

Shearing   Force that occurs when skin moves one way while bone and tissue under the skin move another way.

Sigmoid Colon   Lower portion of the large intestine which curves in an 'S' shape.

Skin Integrity   Unbroken; normal skin.

Smooth Muscle Tissue   Involuntary muscle tissue.

Social Needs   Basic human need for approval and acceptance.

Social Security Act   Act of 1935 providing income to people aged 65 and over.

Spasm   Involuntary contraction of muscle.

Sphincter   Type of muscle that contracts to close a body opening.

Spinal Cord   Long cable of nerves that extends from below the medulla to the second or third lumbar vertebra.

Spiritual   Relates to religious matters or the supranatural.

Spontaneous Combustion   Ignition of burnable materials caused by a chemical reaction.

Sputum   Mucus from the lungs, usually mixed with saliva.

Staphylococcus   Type of harmful bacteria commonly found in health care institutions; treated by antibiotic drugs.

Stasis   Stoppage of flow.

Sterile   Free from all microorganisms.

Sterilization   Process of killing all microorganisms.

Steroids   Drugs used for inflammatory conditions.

Stimulus   Action or agent that causes a response in an organ or organism.

Stool   Solid waste material discharged from the body through the rectum and anus; feces, excreta, excrement, bowel movement, fecal material.

Streptococcus   Type of harmful bacteria commonly found in health care institutions; treated by antibiotic drugs.

Stress   Tension of the mind and in body.

Striated Muscle Tissue   Type of voluntary muscle tissue.

Stringent Strict.

Subcutaneous Below the skin.

Subjective Observations Individiual judgments based on personal feelings.

Subservient Inferior to or below another.

Superior Toward the head.

Supination To turn palms up.

Susceptibility Lack of ability to resist disease.

Sweat Glands Glands that produce moisture to cool the body and excrete waste products.

Tact Ability to say or do the right thing at the right time.

Tardive Dyskinesia Involuntary movements of tongue, facial muscles, fingers and toes due to some medications.

Tendon Elastic cord-like structure that connects muscle to bone.

Testosterone Male hormone.

Territoriality A claim for possession of the area or an object.

Therapeutic Pertaining to or effective in treatment or recovery.

Theory A belief about a set of facts.

Thrombus Blood clot.

Thymus Gland Two-lobe ductless gland believed to play a role in the immune system of the body.

Thyroid Gland Largest of the endocrine glands; secretes thyroid hormone.

Tissue Group of the same type of cells functioning in the same way.

Tolerance The ability to continue in the present state.

Toxins Waste products released by disease-producing organisms.

Traction Exertion of "pull" by means of weights.

Trachea Windpipe; the passage that conveys air from the larynx to the bronchi.

Tracheostomy Opening in the windpipe.

Transfer To move from one place to another.

Trust Believing another person is truthful and can be relied on for support and faithfulness.

Tumor A swelling or enlargement.

Tympanic Membrane Thin membrane inside the ear that vibrates when struck by bound waves; the eardrum.

Tuberculosis Infectious disease which most commonly affects the respiratory system.

Ulcer Break in the skin or mucosal lining creating an open wound.

Ulnar Deviation Away from the thumb side of the hand.

Universal Precautions Using goggles, gloves, gowns, and masks and using other precautions appropriately when handling blood and other body fluids.

Ureters Tubes that extend from the kidneys to the bladder through which urine passes.

Urethra Tube from the bladder to the outside of the body.

Urinary Incontinence Inability to control urination.

Vaginitis Inflammation of the tissue of the vagina.

Vascular Refers to blood vessels.

Veins Blood vessels that carry blood back to the heart.

Venules Very tiny veins that carry blood from the capillaries to the large veins.

Vertebrae Special bones of the spine.

Villi Small finger-like projections of the duodenum which absorb digested food particles and release them into the bloodstream.

Virus Microorganism that can cause infection and disease.

Vital Signs Temperature, pulse, blood pressure, and respiration.

Vulvitis Inflammation of the vulva.

INDEX

Abdominal thrusts, 190–93 (*See also* Heimlich maneuver)
Abduction, 162–66
Abuse, 6
Accidents, 129–33
  factors contributing to, 130
  monitoring, 131
  preventing, 130
Activities of daily living, 36
Acute, infection, 118
Age-related changes (*See* Aging process)
Aging, 19–38
  changes and consequences, 19–38
  emotional aspects, 37
  psychosocial aspects of, 37
Aging process, physiological changes, 19–38
Agitation, coping with, 233
AIDS, 122
Airway obstruction, 189–200
Alzheimer's disease, 228–38
Ambulation, 132
  checklists for, 132–33
  devices for, 75
Anatomy:
  circulatory system, 21–23
  digestive system, 28–29
  endocrine system, 30–31 (*See also* Glands)
  integumentary system, 20
  musculoskeletal system, 25–26
  nervous system, 36
  reproductive system, 33–34
  respiratory system, 22
  urinary system, 31–32
Aneurysm, 244
Angina, definition of, 265
Aphasia, 243
Arrest, cardiac, 267
Arteries, major, 23
Arteriosclerosis, 21
Arthritis, 255
Asepsis:
  medical, 116
  surgical, 116
Asthma, 261
Atherosclerosis, 264–65
Atrophy, muscular, 25

Automobile, transfers, 175

Back strain, avoiding, 28–30
Bacteria, 116–17
  harmful, 117
Bathing, dying resident, 294
Baths:
  paraffin, 258
  whirlpool, 258
Bed, positioning residents in, 157–60
Behavior, in dementia:
  agitation, 233
  hallucination, 233
  sundowning syndrome, 232
  wandering, 233
Bill of Rights, resident's, 6
Bladder management, 215–17
Blood:
  and body fluid precautions, 122
  vessels, 23
Body alignment (*See* Positioning residents in bed)
Body fluid precautions, blood and, 122
Body mechanics, 156
Body system (*See* Anatomy)
Body temperature (*See* Temperature)
Bomb threat, 147
Bones, names of, 27
Bowel management, 217–18
  elimination, reporting and charting, 225
  incontinence, 218
  retraining, 218
Brain:
  Alzheimer's disease, 231
  anatomy, 36
Breathing, obstructed, 189–200
Bronchitis, 261
Burns, preventing, 66

Calories, need for, 182
Cancer, geriatric nursing assistant responses, 254
Cardiac arrest, signs of, 268–69
Cardiac emergencies, 267
Cardiopulmonary resuscitation (*See* CPR)

Cardiovascular system, geriatric nursing assistant responses, 21–22 (*See also* Circulatory system)
Caregiver:
　checklist, 7–9
　description, 7
Cartilage, 256
Casts, geriatric nursing assistant responses, 305
Cataracts, 57
Catheters:
　in-dwelling, 245
　infections due to, 119
Cells, theories of changes, 18
Center of gravity, 130
Cerebral vascular accident, geriatric nursing assistant responses, 245 (*See also* Strokes)
Charting, 105–6
Chemotherapy, side effects of, 253
Choking, 189–200
Chronic obstructive pulmonary disease, 260
Circulatory system, 21–22
　geriatric nursing assistant responses, 21–22
Cognitively impaired, 228
Communicable conditions, 117
Communication:
　barriers, 98–99
　checklists for, 98, 104
　elements of, 96
　humor, 103–4
　non-verbal, 97–98
　telephone, 106–7
　touch, 101–3
　written, 105–6
Compensations:
　for hearing losses, 59–64
　for loss of sensation in fingers and toes, 66
　for sensitivity to heat and cold, 65–66
　for visual losses, 48–59
Conduct, checklist for, 15–16
Confidentiality, 96–97
Confusion, 48
Congestive heart failure, 265
Constipation, 217–18
Contaminated articles, handling, 120
Coordination, muscular, 161–67
CPR, 268–70
Critical time, admission, 86–87
Crying, coping with, 243

Death:
　care of the body after, 296
　physical signs of, 293
Decubiti, 245
Dehydration (*See* Fluid balance)
Dementia:
　irreversible, 229
　reversible, 229
Depression, 239
Devices:
　ambulation, 75
　assistive feeding, 246
Diabetes:
　care of the resident with, 249–50
　reactions in, 250
Diagnostic related groups, 86
Diet:
　special, 187
　well-balanced, 182
Digestive system, 28–30

geriatric nursing assistant responses, 187
Dining rooms, 76
Disabilities, coping with, 227
Disaster preparedness, 140
Diseases:
　Alzheimer's, 228
　arthritis, 255
　asthma, 261
　cancer, 252
　cardiovascular, 264–65
　communicable, 117
　diabetes mellitus, 247
　respiratory, 261
Dissatisfied behavior, coping with, 86–87
Diverticulum, 184
Double bagging, 126
Dressing self, devices for, 245
Drop attacks, 130
Drugs, reactions to, 309
Dying residents:
　caregiver coping, 289
　caring for, 293–94
Dying, stages of, 288

Ears, changes in, 59–61
Eating devices, assistive, 246
Eating, restorative programs for, 245
Elderly:
　classifications of, 1–2
　definition of, 1
　nutrition and the, 182–85
　sex and the, 33
　special needs of the, 38–40
Elderly population, 2
Electricity, safety with, 78
Elimination:
　geriatric nursing assistant responses, 217
　reporting and charting, 217
Embolus, 244
Emergencies:
　cardiac, 267
　respiratory, 262
Emphysema, 261
Employee responsibilities, 16
Endocrine system, 30–31
Enemas, position for, 160
Environment, 74–78
　adjustments, 81–83
　checklist for, 81–83
　effects of, 74
　humanizing, 94
　needs of, 74
Ethical responsibilities, 5
Exercises:
　range of motion, 161–67
　respiratory, 261
Extremities, changes in, 66
Eyes, changes in, 48–58

Facilities, organizational chart, 4
Families:
　feelings of with Alzheimer's, 237–38
　grieving, 289
　helping with admission, 87
　involvement, 82
Fecal impaction, 218
Feeding:
　assistive, 246
　blindness, 59
　gastrostomy, 205
　guidelines for feeding residents, 188–89
　tube, 203
Fiber, in diets, 185

Finger sweeps, 196
Fire, major causes of, 140
Fire safety, 140–45
Fluid:
  balance, intake and output, 185
  imbalance, 185
Fluids:
  geriatric nursing assistant responses, 201–2
  intravenous, 200
Food groups, basic, 183
Food intake, calculating and recording, 209
Fractures, bone, 28

Gait belt, 132
Gastrostomy (*See* Feeding)
Geriatric:
  healthcare team, 2–3
  nurse practitioner, 3
  nursing assistant, description, 3
  nursing assistant prerequisites, 9
Glands, endocrine, 30–31
Glaucoma, 56
Gloves, donning and removing, 127
Gown, isolation, donning and removing, 125
Grief, stages, 288

Handwashing, 121–22
Health care:
  plan, characteristics of, 4
  team, 2–3
Hearing, 59–61
  aids, 62
  losses, 59–61
Heart, 22
Heart attacks, signs and symptoms of, 264–65
Heart disease, geriatric nursing assistant responses, 267
Heart failure, congestive, 265
Heimlich maneuver, 190
Hernia, hiatal, 28
High blood pressure (*See* Hypertension)
Hip, external rotation of, 166
Holistic care, 9
Home health care, 3
Homeostasis, 325
Hormones (*See* Endocrine; Glands)
Hospice care, 295
Human immunodeficiency virus, 122
Humanistic (*See* Philosophy of geriatric nursing care)
Humor (*See* Communication)
Hyperglycemia, 248–49
Hypertension, 264
Hyperthermia, 65
Hypoglycemia, 248–49
Hypothermia, 65

Imbalance, fluid, 185
Impaction, fecal, 218
Incidents:
  log, 131
  reporting, 134
Incontinence:
  bowel, 218
  urinary, 216
Independence, promoting, 5
Infection, 115–123
  susceptibility to, 118–20
  transmission of, 119
Injuries, checklist for preventing, 130
Insulin, reactions to, 249

Integumentary system, 19–20
  age-related changes, 19
  geriatric nursing assistant responses, 19
Interpersonal skills, developing, 93–94
Intravenous fluids, 200–2
  geriatric nursing assistant responses to, 201–2
Isolation, residents in, 123
Isolation gown, 125
Isolation technique, 123–28
Isolation unit, 123–28

Job description, geriatric nursing assistant, 7
Joints, swollen or painful, 257

Kidneys, 32
Knots, tying, 137
Kyphosis, 25

Levels of need, 38–39
Licensed practical nurse, 3
Lifting, guidelines for, 169
Lifting and moving residents, 168
Ligament, 256
Line of gravity, 130
Listening skills (*See* Communication)
Lordosis, 28

Macular degeneration, 57
Maslow's hierarchy of needs, 38–39
Meals, serving, 186
Mealtimes, preparing for, 187–88
Mechanical lift, 169
Medicare act, 86
Microorganisms, 116–17
Modified diets (*See* Diet)
Moving and lifting residents, 169–172
Multi-infarct dementia, 238
Muscular system, 25–28
  geriatric nursing assistant responses, 28
Myocardial infarction, 265–66

Nails, trimming, precautions, 250
Nasal cannula, 302
Nasogastric tube, 203
  feedings, 203
Needs:
  Maslow's hierarchy of, 38–39
  total person, 38–40
Nervous system, 36–37
Neurons, 36
Nosocomial, 118
Nursing care:
  basic, 7
  team, 3
Nursing department, hierarchy chart of, 4
Nutrition, 181–87
  basic, 183
  special, 187

Organizing your time, 329
Orientation, loss of (*See* Confusion)
Osteoarthritis, 257
Osteoporosis, 25
Oxygen, safety precautions for, 303
Oxygen therapy, 301
  checklist for, 303–4

Paralysis, 243
Paraplegics, 243
Parkinson's disease, 238
Pathogenic organisms, 116
Perineal care, 33

Personal qualities, desirable, 9
Philosophy of geriatric nursing care, 9–10
Pick's disease, 238
Plan of care, 40
Pneumonia, 119
  hypostatic, 156
Population, elderly, 2
Positioning, residents in bed:
  Fowler's, 159
  prone, 157
  semiprone, 158
  semisupine, 158
  Sims', 160
Postural:
  drainage, 263
  support, 135–36
Presbycusis, 59
Pressure sores, 156
Preventing accidents, 130
Priorities, setting, 329
Privacy, importance of, 74
Professional registered nurse, 3
Prostate gland, 32
Protective devices, 136
Pseudodementia (*See* Depression)
Psychosocial aspects of aging, 37
Pulse, radial measuring, 156

RACE, fire safety, 145
Radial pulse, 156
Radiation therapy, side effects of, 253
Range of motion exercises, 161–67
Rapport, 96
Reality orientation, 235–36
Rectum (*See* Digestive system)
Rehabilitation:
  geriatric health care team, 2
  professionals who contribute to, 3–4
Relationships:
  employee-employer, 8–9
  foundations, 96–97
  therapeutic, 93
Religious beliefs, observing, 294
Reporting:
  objective, 97–99
  subjective, 97–99
Reproductive system:
  age-related changes in, 33
  geriatric nursing assistant responses,
    33–36
Rescue procedures:
  blanket pull, 146
  two-person carry, 147
Respirations, observing, 262
Respiratory:
  diseases, 261
  emergencies, 262
Respiratory system:
  age-related changes in, 24–25
  effects of immobility, 156
Responsibilities, legal and ethical, 5
Restraints, protective, 135
Rheumatoid arthritis, 257
Role changes, 37

Senses, 48–66
Sensory losses (*See* Senses)
Sensory system (*See* Senses)
Skeletal system (*See* Muscular system)
Skin (*See* Integumentary)
Smell, sense of, 64–65
Smoking, effects of, 260
Social, changes, 37
Social Security Act, 1

Sores, pressure, 156
Spiritual needs, 39
Sputum, in respiratory disease, 262
Stages of dying, Kübler-Ross, 288
Staphylococcus, 119
Stool, check for, 218
Stress, 323–29
  coping, 326–27
  plan for control, 332–33
  reactions to, 325
  stressors, 327–28
  test, 326
Strokes, 243–46
  nursing care of residents with, 244
Suicide, 240
Sundowning syndrome, 232
Surgery, in cancer, 253
Systems, body (*See* Anatomy)

Tactile, compensation for, 78
Taste, sense of, 64–65
Team, health care, 4
Telephone, communications, 106–7
Temperature, conditions of:
  hyperthermia, 65
  hypothermia, 65
  measuring, need for, 65, 262
Territoriality, 74
Theories of aging:
  cross link, 18
  free-radical, 18
  immunological, 18
  programmed aging, 18
Thrombus, 244
Time management:
  daily time manager, 331
  worksheet, 329
Tongue-jaw lift, 196
Touch:
  communication technique, 101
  guidelines for using, 103
Tracheostomy, 300
Traction, 306
Transfer:
  belt, 132
  checklists for, 132–33
  techniques, 168–72
Transporting residents, 173–74
Trapeze, 307
Trust, 97
Tub baths, for arthritis, 258
Tube feedings, 203–6
Tubes, residents with, 202
Turning residents, 156

Unconscious choking victim, 194–200
Universal precautions, 122–23
Urinary, problems, 215–17
Urinary system, 31–33
  age-related changes in, 31–33
  measuring output of, 209
  nursing measures related to, 33

Veins, major, 23
Vessels, blood, 23
Visual losses, 48–58
Vocabulary, in Alzheimer's disease,
  234–35

Walking (*See also* Ambulation)
Wandering, 233
Wheelchairs, transferring to, 169–72
Whirlpool baths, 258